Heal the GUT

Heal the IMMUNE SYSTEM

Scott A. Johnson

Heal the gut, heal the immune system / Scott A. Johnson

ISBN-13: 979-8988720614

Discover more books by Scott A. Johnson at authorscott.com

Published by Scott A. Johnson Professional Writing Services, LLC: Orem, UT

In gratitude to my loving Heavenly Father who has blessed me with the talents and drive to research health and natural solutions so I can write books for the benefit of my fellow man. Years ago, He redirected my life with the diagnosis of a chronic illness and called me to a greater path that has been extremely fulfilling.

Contents

1

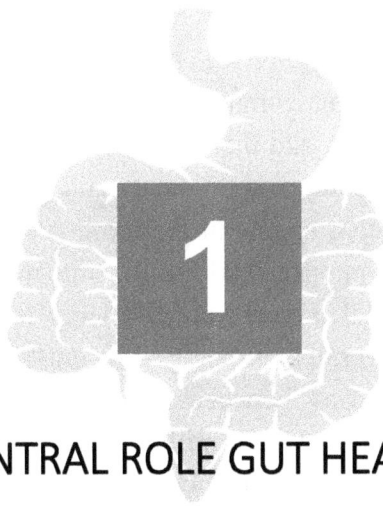

THE CENTRAL ROLE GUT HEALTH PLAYS IN HUMAN HEALTH

Gut health—the health and function of the gastrointestinal (GI) tract from the mouth to intestines—is central to human health. It is responsible for the digestion and absorption of nutrients from food, has its own nervous system (enteric nervous system), houses roughly 70 percent of the immune system (gut-associated lymphoid tissue), and contains trillions of microorganisms that collectively make up the gut microbiome. The gut not only is responsible for digestion, but also aids key body functions such as immunity, hormone regulation, and mood state. Indeed, ample evidence now exists to demonstrate that your gut microbiome and barrier, or integrity of the GI tract, are the major keys to gut health, and substantially impact overall health at any age.[1,2]

Your gut influences everything from inflammation to mood, blood sugar levels to back pain, and can even be the root cause of many health conditions. Compromised gut health leads to many issues throughout the body, including autoimmune and autoinflammatory conditions. Maintaining gut health, which optimizes metabolism and helps maintain a healthy inflammatory response, is absolutely essential for improving your mental, emotional, and physical well-being. Everyone needs to understand the importance of gut health because your entire well-being depends on how well it functions.

The Gut-Brain Axis

Research shows that the gut communicates with the brain through neurotransmitters, hormones, and the vagus nerve—also known as the tenth cranial nerve; comprising the main nerves of your parasympathetic system that begins in the brain (medulla oblongata), extending down through your neck and splitting into many branches that connect to vital abdominal organs—about energy levels, mood, and other factors that affect overall well-being.[3] The gut-brain axis is a two-way communication pathway between the GI tract and the central nervous system involving nearly 500 million gut neurons (nerve cells). It is a signaling channel by which the food we eat transmits information to the brain after being broken down by digestive enzymes and acted upon by bacteria present in the gut. This interaction significantly shapes our moods, cognition, stress responses, memories, and even how the brain ages. The gut-brain axis connects intestinal functions with the emotional and cognitive centers of the brain. Rather than working independently and dominating the control of body functions, modern science reveals that feedback back into the brain from organs like the gut dramatically impacts body functions. Gut-brain communication is strongly influenced by the microbes present in your gut.

Metabolites produced by gut microbes, like short-chain fatty acids (butyrate, propionate, and acetate), can cross the blood-brain barrier and impact the brain's structure and function.[4] Short-chain fatty acids are byproducts produced in the colon when gut microbes ferment dietary fibers and resistant starches. Studies demonstrate that levels of short-chain fatty acids change in many neurological diseases, including Alzheimer's disease, Parkinson's disease, multiple sclerosis, autism spectrum disorder, stroke, and depression.[5] Your gut even produces neurochemicals like GABA and serotonin (90 percent of serotonin is produced in the gut) that affect nervous system function.[6] An intricate connection between the gut and brain partly explains why you might feel "butterflies in your stomach" when nervous or excited and a "hangry" mood when you are hungry. The more we learn about your "second brain," the more we find that the gut significantly influences neural, immune, and endocrine function, and its dysregulation participates in the initiation and progression of multiple diseases.

Your Microbiome

Your body is full of trillions of microbes—bacteria, archaebacteria, viruses, fungi, and other microscopic living things—collectively known as the microbiome. These microbes, and therefore a microbiome, exist in the gut, skin, mouth, nasal cavities, urogenital system, and even the eyes. Each microbiome is its own ecosystem that is sensitive to temperature, pH, nutrients, toxins, and other environmental influences. The greater the diversity in these microbiomes, the more resilient and adaptable to a changing environment they are. In a way, humans could be considered microbial beings because these microbes in and on the human body and the genes they contain outnumber our own cells. Research suggests that bacterial microbes alone outnumber human cells about 1.3 to 1,[7] and this doesn't even consider the fungi and viruses present in and on our body. Humans have formed a vital and symbiotic relationship with these microbes that has shaped human biology and behavior over millennia.

To demonstrate the power of your microbiomes, we need to understand that each microbiome acts as an organ in a way, communicating chemically with other microbiomes and organs throughout the body. Similar to gut-brain communication, an intricate communication relationship exists between the oral (in the mouth) and gut microbiome, the gut microbiome and respiratory microbiome, the skin microbiome and gut microbiome, and likely many others.[8,9,10,11,12] This communication leads to changes in biological function and activities, but may also shape or reshape the microbial ecosystem in each location. Meaning that the signals your oral microbiome sends your gut microbiome may lead to changes in the composition and diversity of either microbiome. Indeed, crosstalk between the gut microbiome, immune system, and tumor microbiome—yes, even cancerous tumors form unique and divergent microbiomes—may yet have implications in immune responses to and progression of cancer.[13] The interaction between your various microbiomes and the environment and other areas of the body is dynamic and has an enormous impact on human health.

To illustrate how a distant microbiome can affect biological function, we can look at emerging research linking the regular use of over-the-counter alcohol-based mouthwash with diabetes risk. The oral microbiome is the second largest microbial habitat in the human body. Despite this, far less is known about its physiological functions and implications in human health. However, we do know that the oral microbiome can affect oral health, overall health, and the risk of certain systemic conditions.[14,15] This was shown by researchers who evaluated the effects of frequently using an alcohol-based antibacterial mouthwash. What this fascinating research found was that people who used mouthwash twice or more daily had a significantly greater risk of developing prediabetes or progressing from prediabetes to diabetes when compared to those who used it less frequently.[16] The theory is that some mouthwashes may alter the oral microbiome ecosystem and lead to the overgrowth of pathogenic bacteria, unless the mouthwash is more selective in targeting pathogenic bacteria and potentially even acts as a prebiotic (something essential oils may do). Furthermore, bacteria present in the mouth play an important role in the salivary conversion of nitrate and nitrite to nitric oxide, and reduced levels of nitric oxide are associated with insulin resistance and adverse cardiovascular effects.[17] Nitric oxide plays a role in the control and regulation of metabolism, glucose utilization, energy production, and body composition, so disrupting its production in the mouth can have far-reaching effects. Emerging evidence suggests that the oral microbiome plays a diverse and important role in human health beyond plaque and cavities.

While microenvironments of microbes exist throughout the body, the gut microbiome is the most well-studied. Your gut microbiome is first populated while in your mother's womb with the delivery of microbes from the placenta (phase 1).[18,19] When you were a fetus in your mother's womb, you did not live in a sterile environment—you were exposed to the bacteria that traveled from your mother's gut into her bloodstream and passed through the placenta. As you swallowed amniotic fluid now filled with bacteria from your mother's microbiome, these microbes interacted with and colonized your fetal intestinal tract. Further colonization of your microbiome occurred as you passed through the birth canal. Under optimal conditions, a full-term, vaginally delivered newborn ingests a healthy amount of vaginal/colonic bacteria as it travels through the birth canal (phase 2). Those that were born by cesarean section missed out on this exposure to microbes and frequently experience dysbiosis (an imbalance in the gut microbiome, which is associated with a variety of health problems).[20] Fortunately, this can be overcome with supplementation with prebiotics, probiotics, synbiotics, and breastfeeding—optimal gut-microbiome colonization requires exclusive breastfeeding, where possible, for the first four to six months of life.[21] Further stimulation of a newborn's gut microbiome happens during breastfeeding (phase 3), when solid foods are introduced (phase 4), and during the critical development period of eighteen months to three years (phase 5). Breastfeeding contains nutrients and other stimulating factors that trigger proliferation of important bacterial species like *Bacteroides fragilis*, *Bifidobacterium infantis*, and *Lactobacillus acidophilus*.[22] Ideally, infants will also be supplemented with an age-appropriate probiotic.

During childhood, your gut microbiome diversified by adding both numbers and variety of species. Microbiome diversity is an important factor for your health and is arguably most important to establish during childhood development.[23,24] Your core microbiome continues to adapt and change during your lifetime in response to factors like medications, diet, physical activity, stress, sleep, supplementation, and environmental factors.[25] Your microbiome can affect health in many ways and acts as a key interface between your body and your environment. Undeniably, differences in microbiome diversity and health can alter susceptibility to certain illnesses—like diabetes, obesity, cardiovascular disease, neurological disorders, allergies, autoimmune disorders, and inflammatory bowel disease.

The majority of microbes in the gut reside in a pouch of your large intestine called the cecum. The small intestine is usually high in acids, oxygen, and antimicrobials, and the short transit time of food through it makes it more difficult for bacteria to colonize compared to the large intestine. More than 2,100 species of bacteria have been identified in the human gut, with approximately 160 species being common among all humans.[26,27] The gene set of these bacteria is estimated to be about 3.3 million genes—150 times greater than the human genome.[28] Again, we have considerably higher number of microbial genes in our body than we do human genes, adding to the reality that we are microbial beings. Collectively, these microbes weigh between two and five pounds (about the weight of your brain) and essentially function as an extra organ that plays a dramatic role in human health. Remarkably, emerging science reveals that microbes in the gut have a "genetic signature" associated with multiple diseases.[29] In other words, it may be possible to predict your risk of certain illnesses by evaluating bacterial genes present in your microbiome.

Of the thousands of species of bacteria found in the human gut and twelve different phyla (bacterial lineages), more than 90 percent belong to Firmicutes and Bacteroidetes, with meaningful populations of Proteobacteria, Actinobacteria, and Verrucomicrobia.[30,31] Microbiome diversity is strongly associated with the Bacteroidetes-to-Firmicutes ratio. Interestingly, the gut microbiome is not as diverse as microbial communities in other areas of the body, suggesting it has some built-in functional redundancy—the promotion of ecological resilience and stability through different species of microbes having the same or very similar functions to buffer against the loss of a single microbial species. This is similar to a backup generator for when the power goes out. You rely on electricity from the grid, but have an alternate source of electricity that can provide for your needs if necessary.

Modern lifestyles continuously expose the gut microbiome to various stress factors that affect its composition—chlorinated water, food additives, pesticides, heavy metals, antibiotics, pollutants, mycotoxins, medications, and more. These factors could cause harmful long-term changes to the gut microbiome (called dysbiosis), allowing more virulent pathogenic microbes to thrive at the cost of your health.

Emerging research even implies that dysbiosis alters blood-brain barrier function, contributing to brain inflammation.[32] Obviously, this is less than ideal because brain inflammation is linked to anxiety, depression, Alzheimer's, Parkinson's, and other neurological conditions.[33,34] This link with neurological disorders and gut dysbiosis helps explain the connection between antibiotic use and psychiatric disorders.[35] This confirms that factors that shape the gut microbiome can also shape brain function.

Examples of Firmicutes (gram-positive bacteria)

- *Anaerotruncus colihominis*
- *Butyrivibrio crossotus*
- *Clostridium* spp.
- *Coprococcus eutactus*
- *Faecalibacterium prausnitzii*
- *Lactobacillus* spp.
- *Pseudoflavonifractor* spp.
- *Roseburia* spp.
- *Ruminococcus* spp.
- *Veillonella* spp.

Examples of Bacteroidetes (gram-negative bacteria)

- *Bacteroides-Prevotella* Group (*B. vulgatus* & *Prevotella* spp.)
- *Barnesiella* spp.
- *Odoribacter* spp.
- *Porphyromonas* spp.

One maker for dysbiosis is the Bacteroidetes-to-Firmicutes ratio, which is associated with several pathological conditions: obesity, metabolic disorders (type 2 diabetes, nonalcoholic fatty liver disease), and inflammatory conditions. While neither Firmicutes nor Bacteroidetes are good or bad on their own, there are helpful, harmful, and neutral species among both phyla. What's most important is to maintain a healthy balance and diversity of gut flora and the right ratio of each. An optimal ratio is considered 12:620 of Firmicutes to Bacteroidetes.

As your gut microbiome gets out of balance and harbors too many unhealthy bacteria, these bacteria produce endotoxins. Endotoxins are produced by certain gram-negative bacteria and released when they are destroyed. Unfortunately, they don't stay put in the gut, but can pass through the wall of the gut lining into the bloodstream, especially if your leaky gut is more than mild. Once there, endotoxins can bind to TLR4 (toll-like receptor 4) receptors—found on mast cells, immune cells, macrophages, and B lymphocytes—triggering an inflammatory cascade and immune response. One endotoxin produced, called lipopolysaccharide (LPS), can make leaky gut worse by damaging intestinal cells.[36] Maintaining gut microbiome diversity is critical to protect against damage caused by endotoxins.

Your Gut Barrier

The gut is your body's largest interface between you and your external environment. Your GI barrier is more than just a physical barrier. It is a complex functional entity consisting of metabolic functions, immune defenses, and nervous system activity. It is designed to have some permeability for nutrients from food to be absorbed from the GI tract and enter the bloodstream; however, dysbiosis causes the barrier between the gut and the bloodstream to become more permeable (called leaky gut). This allows pathogenic bacteria, toxins, and larger molecules to enter the bloodstream and trigger immune and inflammatory responses. Some microbes even escape the GI tract and travel to organs, such as the liver, leading to organ damage or disease.[37] Leaky gut is virtually omnipresent in modern humans. So, it's not about whether you have it, but about how severe it is. Therefore, leaky gut should be considered on a spectrum from mild to severe since most people have some degree of leaky gut. The complexity of gut function is clear when you understand it must serve two opposite functions simultaneously— the selective permeability of vital nutrients from the GI tract to circulation and preventing the escape of harmful entities like pathogens, antigens, and proinflammatory factors.

One way to view this might be to compare it to a spaghetti strainer. The strainer is your gut barrier, the spaghetti is the larger molecules you don't want to escape out of the gut, and the water is the nutrients your body needs for healthy function. When you strain the water out of your spaghetti, you want the water to escape the strainer, but you don't want to lose the spaghetti down the drain. The challenge for your gut barrier is to allow efficient transport of nutrients across the gut epithelium while rigorously preventing passage of harmful molecules and organisms at the same time. When your gut barrier fails, it would be like drilling larger holes in your spaghetti strainer, which would allow your spaghetti to escape down the drain (into your bloodstream).

Gut-barrier function involves three primary defense mechanisms: 1) a biological barrier comprised of gut flora responsible for fighting colonization by pathogens; 2) an immune barrier containing dendritic cells, T cells, B cells, and macrophages that defends against pathogens; and 3) a mechanical barrier of cells (closed-lining intestinal epithelial cells and capillary endothelial cells) that form tight junctions to restrict the passage of molecules, ions, and cells outside the GI tract. Perhaps Hippocrates was right when he said, "All disease begins in the gut."

In addition to the intrinsic GI barrier of intestinal cells and the tight junctions that tie them together, extrinsic GI barrier components are also a factor in gut integrity. The entire GI tract is coated with mucus created by cells that form the epithelial barrier. Mucus serves as a protective layer against tissue damage and contributes to barrier function in multiple ways. Mucin molecules contain carbohydrates that bind to bacteria and help the GI tract resist colonization and accelerate the clearance of harmful microbes. Diffusion—movement of a substance from an area of high concentration to an area of low concentration until the concentration is nearly equalized in the space—of damaging chemicals is also limited by mucus. Lastly, gastric and duodenal cells produce bicarbonate. Secretion of bicarbonate helps to maintain a neutral pH despite the highly acidic conditions inside the GI tract. This process creates a mucus-bicarbonate barrier that acts as an important first line of defense against gastric acid and pepsin.

Hormones are chemical messengers secreted by the body to modify the function of target cells. Although hormones produced by the endocrine system influence digestive function, the most profound effects are mediated by enteric hormones like gastrin, cholecystokinin, and secretin. Enteric hormones are those produced within the GI tract by the enteric endocrine system, which happens to be the largest endocrine organ in the body. Hormone-secreting cells are dispersed throughout the lining of the stomach and small intestine. They only produce hormones in response to current environmental conditions within the GI tract. Enteric hormones help regulate cellular proliferation in response to injury such as ulceration. Robust control systems within the nervous and endocrine systems coordinate digestive processes.

Six key enteric hormones:
- **Gastrin**: Stimulated by the presence of peptides and amino acids in the GI tract, this hormone promotes the secretion of gastric acid and aids in gastric motility.
- **Secretin**: Produced in response to acidic pH levels, secretin triggers the production of water and bicarbonate from the pancreas and bile duct to help maintain a balanced pH.
- **Ghrelin**: Often called the hunger hormone, ghrelin increases appetite when your stomach is empty.
- **Motilin**: This hormone stimulates your digestive system to help move food from your small intestine to your large intestine, and is involved in the release of insulin and pepsin.
- **Cholecystokinin**: Stimulates the secretion of pancreatic enzymes and bile release from the gallbladder to help digest fats and proteins.
- **Gastric inhibitory polypeptide**: This hormone modestly slows gastric acid secretion and GI tract motility after nutrient ingestion and causes the release of insulin when glucose and fat levels increase in the small intestine.

Prostaglandins are hormone-like lipid compounds that affect several bodily functions, including GI tract health. They decrease stomach acid production and stimulate the release of the protective mucus in the GI tract mentioned above. Prostaglandin E2 and prostacyclin are particularly important for the GI tract because they exert a protective effect for GI cells.

Paneth cells are GI cells that serve to defend against microbes in the small intestine. When exposed to bacteria or bacterial antigens, these cells secrete antimicrobial peptides that help preserve GI barrier function by combating specific bacteria, yeasts, and parasites.

Despite its complex and robust nature, GI barrier function can be disrupted by several potential insults. Exposure to toxins, GI infection by bacteria or viruses, ischemia-reperfusion injury (loss and subsequent return of blood and oxygen supply to the GI tract), transient increases in permeability caused by neutrophil infiltration, stress (which decreases GI mucosal blood flow and alters hormone and cytokine production), and multiple systemic illnesses can cause a breach in GI barrier defenses. Mild breaches can usually be handled and repaired by the body, but massive breaches can be fatal.

The Connection between Ferroptosis and Gut-Immune Health

Just like humans, cells have a life cycle that includes a series of growth and development steps a cell undergoes between its birth (formation by the division of a mother cell), reproduction (division to make two new daughter cells), and death. Cells have several ways they are designed to die and allow new cells to replace them, which can be either regulated cell death or accidental cell death. Programmed cell death allows older cells to voluntarily die in an orderly, sequential manner that does not spill their contents onto surrounding cells and cause damage to them. Although more than thirty cell death models have been identified or proposed, apoptosis, necroptosis, pyroptosis, and senescence are among the most common.[38] Another recently identified type of cell death that is closely related to disrupted immune function is ferroptosis.

Apoptosis: programmed cell death that occurs during cellular growth and development or in response to harmful environmental stimuli.

Necrosis: an umbrella term for a wide variety of premature cell death processes, such as pyroptosis and necroptosis, resulting from cell injury.

Autophagy: death by degradation to eliminate dysfunctional or damaged cellular parts (e.g., organelles and damaged proteins).

Senescence: the cessation of cellular division in response to DNA damage, telomere dysfunction, oncogene activation, or organelle stress.

Entosis: a cellular death process by which one living cell invades or engulfs another cell.

Ferroptosis: programmed cell death dependent on iron whereby iron-dependent peroxidation of lipids in the cell membrane occurs, which results in the accumulation of lipid peroxide.

Ferroptosis has a unique association with iron load inside cells. In essence, imbalance in iron homeostasis inside a cell sparks oxidative stress, exhausts glutathione stores, promotes oxidation of the cell membrane, triggers the failure of intracellular antioxidant systems (glutathione peroxidase, ferroptosis suppressor protein 1, and dihydroorotate dehydrogenase), and ultimately leads to cell death. Ferroptosis has increasingly been associated with neurodegenerative disorders, cancer, cardiovascular disease, traumatic brain injury, and autoimmune conditions.[39,40] Indeed, one of the factors that trigger autoimmunity is abnormal cell death and the inadequate clearance of dead cells, which allows the release of contents inside the cell to activate the immune system and cause inflammatory reactions.

Ferroptosis is likely regulated by microRNAs (miRNAs), histones, and an array of signaling pathway networks. miRNAs are small non-coding molecular compounds important for making functional proteins and the expression of genes. miRNAs regulate ferroptosis by controlling the expression of ferroptosis-related genes and the subsequent accumulation of iron within cells.[41] Histones are proteins that provide structural support for chromosomes. Chromosomes are long chains of DNA wrapped around complexes of histone proteins, making the chromosome take on a more compact shape that fits into the cell nucleus. Histones are also involved in gene expression. Histone modification can alter the binding of regulatory proteins, modify gene expression, affect glutathione production, and resist or promote ferroptosis accordingly. Altering histone interactions with proteins and DNA leads to epigenetic changes that regulate many normal and disease-related processes. Other signaling pathways involved in the regulation of ferroptosis include: adenosine 5′ monophosphate-activated protein kinase (AMPK)—plays a role in ferroptosis related to cellular energy stress; nuclear factor erythroid 2-related factor 2 (NRF2)—plays a role in intracellular iron metabolism and antioxidant responses; tumor suppressor protein p53—slows the depletion of glutathione in cells and the accumulation of reactive oxygen species; and autophagy—closely linked to ferroptosis because autophagic activity is adjusted to promote efficient cellular cleanup in response to ferroptosis and therefore they jointly affect cell death. Understanding how ferroptosis is regulated can lead to the development of clinical strategies that target ferroptosis and the potential to alter the course of diseases associated with it.

Ferroptosis is related to gut health and emerging evidence suggests it plays a role in inflammatory bowel disease (IBD). First, higher incidence of IBD is observed in cultures that have adopted the Western diet rich in highly refined vegetable oils (canola, corn, sunflower, soybean, and rapeseed).[42,43] Curiously, polyunsaturated fatty acids (PUFAs), but not monounsaturated fatty acids (MUFAs)—like palmitoleic acid and oleic acid found in olive and avocado oils—initiate the production of proinflammatory cytokines in intestinal cells.[44] Every time you consume PUFAs, you are providing materials necessary for ferroptosis to occur. Second, small intestine epithelial cells, those that make up the tight junctions of the GI tract, show impaired glutathione peroxidase activity and increased lipid peroxidation in people with

Crohn's disease, both hallmark signs of ferroptosis.[45] Third, a metabolite of gut bacteria called capsiate inhibits ferroptosis, suggesting a role for the gut microbiome in the control of ferroptosis.[46] It not only limits ferroptosis, but also is involved in the expression of proteins and genes that reduce the risk of cardiovascular and musculoskeletal diseases and obesity.[47,48,49] Lastly, animal models demonstrate that dietary factors, like PUFAs, promote ferroptosis and colitis while factors that inhibit ferroptosis alleviate colitis.[50,51] The evidence is becoming more clear that ferroptosis causes dysfunction of the intestinal epithelium, contributing to several intestinal diseases.

2

THE MARVELOUSLY DESIGNED IMMUNE SYSTEM

Your body's natural defense system, the immune system, is made up of an army of special cells, organs, proteins, and tissues designed to protect you against infection and illness every single day. This complex network acts in a coordinated manner, with each component performing specific functions to fight foreign invaders (bacteria, viruses, fungi, parasites, and toxins). We tend to take our immune systems for granted when we are in a state of health but are reminded that it is present when we are sick and it is fighting the cause of that illness. Given the complexity of the immune system, its functions, and interactions with other systems and molecules in the body, the following information will be more technical, but is important to understand in the context of healing the immune system. Your immune system is your best defense against sickness and injury, but when it goes amiss, it can be your worst enemy, causing challenging chronic disorders.

The Innate and Adaptive Immune Systems

The immune system has two parts—innate and adaptive. The innate (nonspecific) immune system is present at birth and acts as your first line of defense against foreign invaders. It relies on a series of nonspecific defenses that guard against all infections, not any one specific pathogen. Like clockwork, it responds the same way to all foreign substances until the second part of your immune system, the adaptive immune system, kicks in. The most important defensive organ of the innate immune system is the skin, which provides a physical barrier to keep pathogens out of the body. Additional defenses are employed if a pathogen enters the body through an opening in the skin, including saliva, mucus, and tears, which contain an enzyme that attacks the cell walls of bacteria. Additionally, an inflammatory response begins that increases blood flow to an infected area, and blood vessels expand, allowing white blood cells to escape from the bloodstream and enter infected tissue. Pathogens that bypass all these innate immune defenses activate the adaptive immune response.

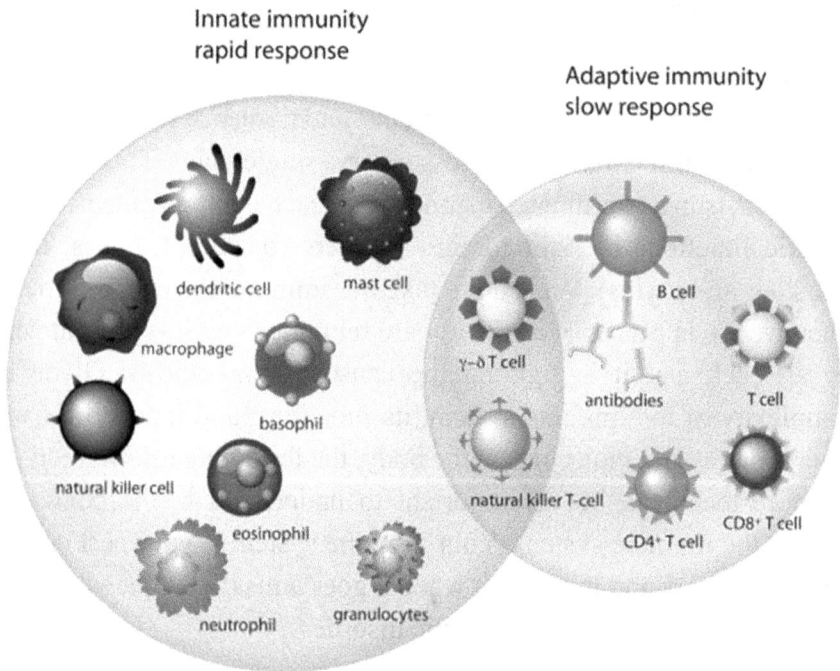

Adaptive, or acquired immunity, is learned as the immune system encounters antigens (chemicals, bacteria, viruses, fungi, parasites, or smaller proteins that pathogens express). Antigens are usually located on the surface of pathogens, with each pathogen having a unique antigen that a corresponding antibody is designed to attack. Once attached to the cells, antibodies recruit cells that will engulf and destroy the pathogen to the area. The adaptive immune system also remembers antigens, which allows your immune system to mount a more rapid and effective response in the case of a subsequent antigen exposure. Your adaptive immune system becomes "smarter" with each antigen it encounters and relies on these encounters to maintain adequate defenses against them.

Adaptive immunity is developed throughout life as the immune system encounters pathogens and creates memory T and B cells in response. These memory cells allow the body to respond to and destroy pathogens that it has previously encountered more rapidly and effectively. Adaptive immunity can also be transferred from mother to baby through antibodies shared between mother and baby during gestation and passed through breast milk.

Types of T cells:

> Killer T cells attach to antigens or abnormal cells and create holes in their membrane for destruction.

> Helper T cells coordinate the efforts of, or aid, other immune cells. They may help B cells produce antibodies or activate killer T cells and macrophages to process infected or abnormal cells.

> Suppressor T cells are responsible for ending the immune response after an antigen is dealt with or inhibiting responses that may be harmful or damage tissues.

B Cells respond to pathogens in two stages:

> *Primary immune response.* Antigens attach to receptors on B cells and differentiate into plasma or memory B cells. The plasma cells produce antibodies, whereas the memory cells remain in the lymph tissue to manage the next encounter with the same antigen. Production of sufficient antibodies generally takes days the first time the B cells encounter the antigen.

» *Secondary immune response.* Once the body has encountered an antigen, memory B cells remember this encounter and change into plasma cells, which multiply and produce antibodies rapidly during subsequent infections. The secondary immune response is much faster.

Antibodies have two parts: 1) a variable part that changes and is specialized to attach to one specific antigen; and 2) a constant part that determines the antibody's class and function and is composed of one of five structures:

»» IgA defends against organisms that enter through surfaces lined with a mucous membrane (digestive tract, nose, eyes, and lungs).

»» IgD is present in the membrane of immature B cells and helps them mature. Scientists don't fully understand its function but know it is involved in the activation of B cells.

»» IgE is involved in immediate allergic reactions and defends against some types of parasites. It binds to basophils and mast cells, which release substances like histamine when they encounter allergens. These substances increase inflammation and damage tissues in the area.

»» IgG is the most common class of antibody and is responsible for defending against bacteria, viruses, fungi, and toxic substances. IgG is able to cross the placenta to the fetus and provides protection for the fetus.

»» IgM is located mainly in the blood and lymph fluid and are the first antibodies to be produced in response to a newly encountered antigen.

Cell-Mediated Immune Response

Cell-mediated immunity is an immune response that leverages the activation of macrophages and natural killer cells (NKCs), the release of cytokines, and the production of antigen-specific cytotoxic T cells in response to an antigen. It does not involve antibody production. As a pathogen enters the body, it frequently encounters cells of the innate immune system, which consume and process the pathogen. These cells then become antigen-presenting cells that carry the pathogen into the lymphatic system for presentation to other immune cells. T cells in the lymphatic tissue are activated in response to this presentation of the pathogen and rapidly spread throughout the body to kill the pathogen and any cells already infected. Some T cells, called memory T cells, remain in the lymphatic tissue for the next time the body is infected with the same pathogen. By responding to subsequent infections by the same pathogen more rapidly, the severity and duration of symptoms can be reduced.

Humoral Immune Response

Humoral immunity is antibody-based and relies on antibodies circulating throughout the body. Antibodies, also called immunoglobulins, are immune proteins that bind to unwanted substances to eliminate them from your body. This response begins when an antibody on a B cell binds to an antigen. After processing the antigen inside the B cell, it presents this antigen to specialized T-helper cells, subsequently activating the B cell. Activated B cells grow rapidly, producing plasma cells and memory B cells to deal with the substance.

> » Plasma B cells produce thousands of antibodies, which are released into the bloodstream and lymphatic system.

> » Memory B cells stay in the lymphatic system and respond to subsequent infections by the same pathogen.

Your body uses several mechanisms to respond to pathogens when they enter the body including the following:

Fever. Although considered a symptom of infection or illness, a fever is actually corrective action being taken by the immune system to create an environment less hospitable for invading organisms. Mild fevers after infection are a good indication that your immune system is functioning well. An elevated body temperature also initiates cellular mechanisms that drive the immune system to act against an offending antigen. Nuclear factor kappa B (NF-κB) is a family of transcription factors that regulate a large array of genes involved in immune and inflammatory processes. These proteins act as a switchboard operator, responding to an antigen by turning relevant genes related to immune responses on and off at the cellular level. Dysregulation of NF-κB is linked to autoimmune and autoinflammatory diseases like rheumatoid arthritis, Hashimoto's, Chron's disease, multiple sclerosis, psoriasis, and Blau syndrome.[52] NF-κB proteins wait inactive in the body, poised to respond when their inhibition is temporarily removed. Multiple mechanisms constrain the activity of these proteins, including mechanisms that terminate their activity once an antigen has been neutralized. Despite a complex regulatory network, NF-κB sometimes disrupts cellular homeostasis, leading to immune disorders. NF-κB plays a key role in the intestinal immune system and restoring balance in its activity is a therapeutic target for chronic inflammatory conditions. You want NF-κB to be active enough for satisfactory protection but restrained enough to not harm healthy cells and tissues.

White Blood Cells. The cells involved in the immune response are white blood cells, or leukocytes, which travel in your bloodstream and pass through vessel walls and tissues to sites of infection or injury. About 60 to 70 percent of white blood cells are produced in bone marrow, while lymphatic tissue (spleen, thymus, and lymph nodes) produce about 20 to 30 percent of white blood cells, and the remaining white blood cells (around 4 to 8 percent) are produced in the reticuloendothelial tissues of the spleen, liver, lymph nodes, and other organs. They are stored in the blood and lymphatic tissues, where they are circulated until called into action.

Types of white blood cells:

> » Lymphocytes are white blood cells that create antibodies in response to foreign invaders that help your immune system fight infections and cancer. There are two primary types of lymphocytes: B lymphocytes (B cells) create antibodies that attack harmful and invading organisms, and T lymphocytes (T cells) control immune responses and directly attack and kill infected cells and

tumor cells. T cells and B cells work together despite having different roles in your immune system.

B cells have receptors on their surfaces where antigens attach. These receptors are like locks, and when the right key fits into the lock, it triggers a response. With antigen exposure, they learn to recognize the different antigens and respond by producing antibodies specific to the antigen they have encountered. B cells are stimulated after an antigen attaches, which causes them to become plasma cells or memory cells. Plasma cells make antibodies specific to the antigen that stimulated it, which then circulate in the bloodstream until they encounter the antigen. Once they encounter the antigen, the antibody binds to the antigen to neutralize it or mark it for destruction by other immune components. It's somewhat like a laser-guidance system that directs a missile (another immune cell) to destroy the targeted cell.

Your immune system puts in a lot of work to fight an infection, so it has an amazing built-in feature to fight the same pathogen during subsequent encounters. This involves memory cells. Memory cells remain in the body and remember the antigen your immune system previously fought so they can quickly make lots of antibodies and stop the infection in its tracks. Remarkably, memory cells can make enough antibodies to get rid of an antigen in about one-third of the time plasma cells take to make sufficient antibodies during the original infection. They are so efficient that you might get rid of the antigen before you even feel sick.

Natural killer cells (NKCs) are lymphocytes in the same family as T and B cells that do not attack pathogens directly. Instead, they destroy infected or cancerous host cells to prevent the spread of infection and cancer. NKCs are essentially activated to destroy your bases (cells) now occupied by the enemy (antigen) so they can no longer be used as operation centers to continue further attacks on healthy cells. They are part of the innate immune response and natural-born killers, meaning they can recognize and attach to infected and cancerous cells as soon as NKCs are formed. They are best known for killing cells infected by a virus and cells displaying early signs of cancer. NKCs constantly patrol the body, unrelentingly evaluating the other cells they come in contact with. Whether or not they kill the cells they encounter depends on a balance of signals received from two types of receptors on their surface, activating and inhibitory. Activating receptors recognize molecules on the surface of infected and cancerous cells, which switches their killing ability on. Once they recognize and attach to these cells, they release enzymes and other substances that damage the outer membranes of cancerous/infected cells to destroy them. Contrarily, healthy cells present molecules (cognate MHC I) that interact with NKC inhibitor receptors that switch off their killing ability.

» Monocytes are large phagocytic (immune cells that engulf and digest pathogens, cancer cells, cellular debris, and foreign substances) white blood cells that can differentiate into macrophages or dendritic cells. They become macrophages when they are moved from the bloodstream to tissues—which they can readily do—in response to infection. Their ability to roam outside the bloodstream gives them greater range to hunt pathogens. They can also release cytokines to communicate with and recruit other cells to the site of infection.

» The most common type of white blood cells are granulocytes. They fight pathogens and heal damaged cells by releasing the contents of their granules (antimicrobial proteins, enzymes, and reactive oxygen species) into the bloodstream during infections, injuries, and allergic reactions. There are four types of granulocytes: neutrophils, eosinophils, basophils, and mast cells.

Neutrophils, or polymorphonuclear leukocytes, are among the first to respond to antigens. They have a very short lifespan, surviving less than twenty-four hours before undergoing self-destruction, which prevents further tissue injury and excess inflammation. They are phagocytic cells that are also considered granulocytes because they contain granules that are highly toxic to bacteria and fungi. Neutrophils release antimicrobial substances and proteases (enzymes) that degrade and kill microbes. After killing a pathogen, some neutrophils activate macrophages to help remove the pathogens. They circulate in the bloodstream until called upon to enter infected or damaged tissues.

Eosinophils primarily combat intestinal parasites, but they may also be involved in the destruction of cancer cells as well as inflammatory and allergic reactions. When activated, they move into affected tissue and secrete inflammatory substances that destroy foreign organisms. Unfortunately, they can cause damage to the body when they get out of control or too many of them are present in tissues. Eosinophilic esophagitis is a classic example of this damage and involves the buildup of eosinophils in the esophagus, which can inflame and injure esophageal tissue, making it difficult to swallow.

Like eosinophils, basophils are most often involved in activity against parasitic infections. However, they play a role in autoimmune diseases, allergic reactions, and inflammation. They are part of the innate immune system and activate when they come in contact with foreign substances, IgE, or by specific signals sent by other cells. They release stored granules, heavily relying on heparin and histamine, when activated, which enhances blood flow and reduces clotting to quickly transport necessary cells and substances to the site of inflammation.

Unlike the previous three white blood cells, basophils do not ingest harmful organisms. Instead, their granules release histamine in response to allergens (antigens that cause allergic reactions), which improves blood flow to the affected tissues. They also release substances that recruit other white blood cells to affected tissues. Activated basophils can also release cytokines (IL-3 and IL-4), potentially shifting Th1/Th2 balance towards Th2. Maintaining a tightly controlled Th1/Th2 balance decreases autoimmunity risk, promotes immune tolerance, and strengthens the ability of the immune system to fight infections.

Located in the mucous membranes and connective tissues, not the bloodstream, mast cells play a role in wound healing, blood vessel function, bone growth, and defense against pathogens through the inflammatory response. They are particularly prominent in body tissues that interact with the external environment, such as the skin, respiratory system, and digestive tract. Activation of mast cells—like when exposed to an allergen or a perceived pathogen—causes them to rapidly release cytokines, proteases, and granules (like histamine and serotonin), which is called degranulation and leads to a powerful inflammatory cascade. When we eat something that is perceived as harmful, mast cells degranulate, which increases fluid secretion, increases muscle contraction in the GI tract (potentially resulting in vomiting or diarrhea), and accelerates the passage of fecal matter through the colon to move the perceived harmful substance out of the body as quickly as possible. A similar protective response occurs in the respiratory tract. Mast cells constrict airways, prompt coughing, promote congestion, and increase mucus production to protect respiratory tract tissues from the provoking substance. Mast cells can even trigger a skin response when food particles exit the GI tract and enter circulation. Once in the bloodstream, the food particles interact with mast cells in the skin and trigger an inflammatory response that causes swelling, redness, hives, rash, or eczema. Mast cells are effectively triggering defensive responses to accelerate clearance of the antigen from the body. Once more, things perceived as symptoms are actually restorative actions being taken by the body for self-protection.

Histamine intolerance is a condition characterized by an intolerance to foods (fermented foods, alcohol, packaged meat, cured meats, aged cheese, legumes, smoked fish, spinach, nuts, dried fruit, avocados, tomatoes, eggplant, and most citrus fruits) that contain histamine. With histamine intolerance, your body has an impaired ability to metabolize histamine because of a deficiency in the GI enzyme diamine oxidase. Without enough of this enzyme, histamine-containing foods are not broken down and absorbed properly in the GI tract. This leads to uncomfortable symptoms like abdominal cramps, abnormal heart rate, fatigue, flushing, headache or migraines, mood disorders, difficulty regulating body temperature, sleep disturbances, nasal congestion, sneezing, trouble breathing, vertigo, nausea, hives, and high blood pressure. So, histamine intolerance originates in the gut. The solution is to reduce consumption or entirely eliminate histamine-containing foods, foods that release histamine (alcohol, bananas, chocolate, dairy, artificial dyes and preservatives, pineapple, tomatoes, strawberries, wheat germ, shellfish, papaya, and nuts), and foods that block diamine oxidase activity (alcohol, black tea, green tea, mate tea, and energy drinks). After this, you should balance stomach acidity and improve digestion by taking a supplement with betaine, hydrochloric acid (HCL), and pepsin.

Typical dosage: betaine hydrochloride + pepsin, as recommended by the product label—typical dosage in supplements ranges are 500–750 mg betaine HCl and 21–162 mg pepsin (sometimes based on FCC units)

Cautions/Contraindications: Duodenal or peptic ulcer

Potential adverse effects: Generally well tolerated, stomach irritation, heartburn, duodenal ulcer or delayed ulcer healing

While the above discussion is only a small summary of the immune system, even that brief outline makes it unequivocally apparent that the immune system is a complex physiological system. It is a system that protects us from internal and external threats daily. With its pivotal role in growth, development, and longevity, it is obviously a system that we want to place high emphasis on keeping it alert and functioning at an optimum level.

Compromised Immune System Function

To be effective, the immune system needs to be able to discriminate between foreign invaders (nonself) and normal parts of the body (self). Self-particles are proteins and other molecules that are part of, or created by, your body. Nonself-particles are not made by your body and can be bacteria, viruses, parasites, pollen, dust, and toxic chemicals. Occasionally, the adaptive immune system gets confused and mistakenly attacks its own healthy tissues and organs—called autoimmunity. Closely related to autoimmunity, autoinflammatory conditions involve dysfunction of the innate immune system that causes immune cells to target the body's own healthy tissues. In addition, immunodeficiency may occur, which is when part of the immune system is missing or not functioning properly. Other immune system disorders are allergies. When allergies occur, the immune system overreacts to a harmless antigen. Lastly, cancers of the immune system may occur when immune cells grow out of control.

Driven by the adaptive immune system, autoimmunity involves the presence of antibodies created by autoreactive B cells and autoreactive T cells targeted against self-particles. These antibodies that target healthy cells are called autoantibodies, of which there are many types. Emerging research suggests that even healthy people frequently have autoantibodies present in their body, but not all manifest the symptoms associated with those particular antibodies.[53,54] In other words, you may have autoantibodies for an autoimmune thyroid disorder (or any other autoimmune disorder) but have no symptoms of Hashimoto's or Graves' disease (or another autoimmune disorder) the autoantibodies normally cause. This new research suggests that autoimmune conditions may require the autoantibodies to bind with and form complexes with autoantigens—self-antigens made by your body that cause your immune system to attack healthy cells they shouldn't. Without forming these complexes, some common autoantibodies present in healthy individuals remain benign and do not cause symptoms or disease. An autoimmune condition develops when enough of these complexes are present in the body to alter the function of, or damage, healthy organs and tissues. Several types of autoimmune conditions exist, including rheumatoid arthritis, systemic lupus erythematosus, alopecia areata, psoriasis, scleroderma, Sjogren's syndrome, Crohn's disease, Hashimoto's, Grave's disease, type 1 diabetes, multiple sclerosis, and many more. While our lives depend on the complex surveillance network in the immune system, under certain circumstances, it can become hyperactive and identify our own tissues as foreign and target them for destruction.

In autoimmune conditions, autoreactive lymphocytes proliferate polyclonally (descending from two or more cells of different ancestry or genetic makeup) because of immune dysregulation. This means that there are many different types of autoreactive lymphocytes, rather than exact copies of the same lymphocyte. Consider this from the perspective of a painting class. Each student in the class aims to duplicate the painting created by the instructor at the front of the class. However, at the end of the class, each painting will resemble the others but not be an exact duplicate because each student has different artistic skills and talents. Similarly, autoreactive lymphocytes have similar features but contain different antigen receptors on their surface, making them have different cellular targets. Polyclonal proliferation is a distinguishing characteristic between autoimmunity and malignancies that proliferate monoclonally (identical copies of the original cell).

Less recognized and understood, autoinflammatory conditions share similar characteristics with autoimmune conditions but involve a different part of the immune system—the innate immune system. They are characterized by mutations in proteins involved in innate immune responses—NLRP3 inflammasome (mediates proinflammatory responses and contributes to chronic pain), cytokine receptors, and receptor antagonists. Oxidative stress, mitochondrial dysfunction, and protein misfolding also play roles. In autoinflammatory conditions, systemic inflammation is present, but there is a lack of autoantibodies, and the adaptive immune system is not attacking healthy cells. Instead, the innate immune system activates an assault on healthy tissues by triggering the release of chemicals involved in the inflammatory cascade. Once initiated, this assault gets stuck in perpetual assault mode and does not resolve like it should. Types of autoinflammatory conditions include ankylosing spondylitis, familial Mediterranean fever, TNF-receptor associated periodic syndrome (TRAPS), Muckle-Wells, neonatal-onset multisystem inflammatory diseases (NOMID), and others.

Autoinflammatory conditions often have a genetic association and strong family history. But some may be driven by somatic mutations, IL-1-family cytokines (inflammasomes), defective interferon production and signaling, dysregulated nuclear factor kappa-light-chain-enhancer of activated B cells (NFκB) and/or tumor necrosis factor

(TNF) activity, or other inflammatory mechanisms.[55] Somatic mutations involve changes in DNA sequences of any biological cell of the body other than a gamete, germ cell, gametocyte, or undifferentiated stem cell that alter tissues after conception. Better explained, somatic mutations are mutations that were not passed to you from your parents (germline mutations). This means these mutations also do not pass on to offspring. Somatic mutations increase production of proinflammatory molecules and can affect your health or cause autoinflammatory conditions. Inflammasomes are molecules of the innate immune system responsible for the activation of inflammatory responses. Because of this role in inflammation, inflammasome activity must be tightly controlled. Loss of inflammasome control triggers inflammatory responses in macrophages that leads to chronic inflammation and the subsequent development and progression of autoinflammatory conditions. A group of proteins released by cells in response to viruses, interferons—type I interferons (IFN-α and -β)— and interferon signaling are strongly implicated in the development of autoinflammatory conditions. Interferons stimulate immune responses that can trigger the maturation and activation of myeloid dendritic cells. Myeloid dendritic cells act as messengers between the innate and adaptive immune systems. Their main function is to process an antigen and then present it on their surface so T cells can detect it and respond appropriately. By doing so, they promote alterations in Th1/Th2 balance and activate B cells triggering a systemic inflammatory cascade, exposing their underlying roles in autoinflammatory conditions. TNF is a major inflammatory cytokine that activates NFκB in response to a variety of stimuli. Abnormal activation of these signaling pathways disrupts immune homeostasis and induces a systemic inflammatory response. The type of autoinflammatory condition that develops is largely driven by which one or more of these mechanisms is involved in the condition combined with a genetic predisposition.

Immunodeficiency is a state characterized by a weakened or absent immune system that reduces the body's ability to fight infections and cancer. Not surprisingly, about one-quarter of people who are immunocompromised also have an autoimmune disorder. When the immune system strays from homeostasis, rogue cells and signaling molecules can wreak havoc on body tissues. Most cases of immune deficiency are acquired and affect the adaptive immune system. A person with a compromised immune system is more susceptible to infection, experiences more severe illness when sick, stays sick for longer, and gets sick more often.

Primary immunodeficiency is usually present at birth and can be inherited or develop spontaneously. It can occur because of genetic mutations and is classified according to the part of the immune system that is deficient: humoral immunity (B cells), cellular immunity (T cells), both humoral and cellular (B and T cells), phagocytes, or complement proteins (proteins that aid immune responses to bacteria and foreign cells). In contrast, secondary immunodeficiency is caused by an environmental or lifestyle factor, such as an accident that damages the spleen, or medications like those used for cancer treatment. It can even be the result of diabetes since white blood cells do not function well when blood sugar levels are elevated.

Allergies occur when your immune system activates in response to something that doesn't trigger the same response in most people. The offending substance can be pollen, food, mold spores, dust mites, pet dander or hair, insect bites/stings, or medicines. For instance, your immune system may mistakenly identify harmless pollen as a threatening foreign invader and respond by producing antibodies called Immunoglobulin E (IgE). Each type of IgE is specific to a type of allergen, which is why some people are only allergic to cow's milk— because they only have IgE specific to cow's milk in their body—while others are allergic to multiple substances because they have many types of IgE in their body. IgE travels to immune cells (mast cells and basophils) that release chemicals (like histamine, proteases, chemotactic factors) and create other mediators (such as prostaglandins, leukotrienes, platelet-activating factor, cytokines), causing an allergic reaction. The result is the characteristic symptoms of the nose, lungs, sinuses, throat, ears, stomach, and skin.

Common allergic disorders include allergic asthma, eczema, rhinitis, hay fever, conjunctivitis, hives, and food allergies. A combination of genetic and environmental factors likely cause allergies.

Sometimes, cancers—lymphoma, leukemia, and myeloma—of the immune system occur. All of these are cancers that originate in blood cells and can spread throughout the body. With these types of cancer, the cancer cells are not only evading detection by the immune system, but also affecting how the immune system works against other illnesses.

Lymphoma begins in the lymph system, which is a series of vessels and nodes throughout the body. The two major types of lymphoma include Hodgkin lymphoma and non-Hodgkin lymphoma. The primary difference between the two lymphomas is the type of lymphocytes each involves. Hodgkin lymphomas involve a specific type of cell called Reed-Sternberg cells. If the Reed-Sternberg cell is not present, the cancer is non-Hodgkin lymphoma.

Leukemia begins in the bone marrow, where blood cells are made. There are four major subtypes of leukemia: 1) acute lymphocytic leukemia, 2) chronic lymphocytic leukemia, 3) acute myeloid leukemia, and 4) chronic myeloid leukemia. Diagnosis of one type or another depends on how quickly the cancer grows and in which blood cell type it originates. Acute types affect very young white blood cells and generally grow very rapidly. Chronic leukemias impact more mature cells and grow more slowly. Additionally, lymphocytic leukemias affect lymphocytes. If the leukemia affects any other type of blood cell, it is called myeloid leukemia.

Cancer originating in plasma B cells is called myeloma. When plasma cells become cancerous, they multiply and produce abnormal antibodies called M proteins. These cancerous cells may also crowd out healthy blood cells, leading to anemia, peripheral neuropathy, bone loss or damage, kidney problems, or more frequent infections. Four main subtypes of myeloma are recognized: multiple myeloma, plasmacytoma, localized myeloma, and extramedullary myeloma.

Gut Health and Immune Function

Vast amounts of research and clinical experience make the influence the gut has on the immune system undeniable. To start with, the largest part of your immune system is found in your gut, so it goes without saying that immune health follows gut health. Humans and microorganisms have been interdependent for millennia and human immune system function has adapted with and been shaped by these microorganisms.[56,57] The trillions of bacteria and viruses present in the gut are crucial for the maintenance of appropriate immune responses.[58,59,60] A symbiotic and coordinated relationship between the gut microbiome and the immune system is maintained to promote immune homeostasis. Anything that disrupts this delicate balance can cause an immune and inflammatory cascade leading to autoimmune, autoinflammatory, allergic, and skin diseases.

The gut barrier plays a critical role in immunity by defending against the escape of immune-modifying molecules from the GI tract to the bloodstream. An intense communication link between epithelial cells that make up the GI barrier, the microbiome, and immune cells shapes specific immune responses and significantly influences immune balance and tolerance.[61] What happens in the gut not only impacts GI inflammation and intestinal health, but also affects the susceptibility to a range of health conditions.

This leads us into the next aspect of gut-immune health, which is the gut-brain axis. Several neuropeptides (calcitonin gene-related peptide, pituitary adenylate cyclase-activating polypeptide, corticotropin-releasing hormone, and phoenixin) coordinate immune-gut communications that promote immune homeostasis.[62] Neurons and immune cells in the gut communicate to coordinate critical physiological functions and immune responses while healthy and during infection, food allergy, and more. Indeed, gut neurons play a crucial role in regulating the functions of innate immune cells, adaptive immune cells, and intestinal cells.

Evolving research suggests that ferroptosis plays a critical role in immune cell function.[63] What the research has found is that ferroptosis influences lymphocytes, macrophages, neutrophils, NKCs, and dendritic cells. Ferroptosis fundamentally affects immune cells in two ways: it changes the number and function of immune cells, and cells that have undergone ferroptosis are recognized by immune cells, triggering a range of inflammatory or specific response. The balance between cell survival and cell death is critical for human health and homeostasis, and also important for immune function. Disproportionate ferroptotic demise of immune cells may compromise immune responses to infections, harmful invaders, or cancers. On the other hand, ferroptosis in nonimmune cells releases damaged cellular components (called damage-associated molecular patterns) that alert immune cells, increase inflammation, and change immune activity. Excessive or deficient ferroptosis is linked to a growing list of physiological and pathophysiological processes involving a dysregulated immune response.

As humans develop, age, and live life, our immune systems adapt and change accordingly, fine-tuning an intricate equilibrium that provides us with a discerning defense system. Doing so is critical so that the army of immune cells present in the human body can efficiently handle dangerous invaders without heavy casualties to healthy cells and tissues. With a fundamental understanding of gut and immune health and armed with the knowledge that they are closely connected, we can now focus on solutions that emphasize healing the gut to health the immune system.

3

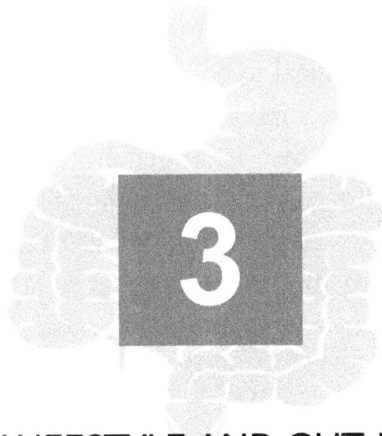

A HEALTHY LIFESTYLE AND GUT-IMMUNE HEALTH

Healing the gut, and therefore the immune system, requires a focus on four key areas: 1) cleansing, 2) strengthening, 3) restoring, and 4) protecting. In reality, healing the gut will improve your overall health and quality of life. Like all things health, there isn't one single solution that is going to promote healing, rather healing necessitates a holistic approach that includes lifestyle adjustments and targeted supplementation.

You Are What You Eat

When homes are built, a strong foundation is laid first. This ensures that the walls and everything built on top of that are functional and sturdy. Similarly, health has a foundation, and it is nutrition. You are what you eat is more than a metaphor—it is a literal fact. The food you eat and drinks you consume are metabolized by the body and the nutrients (both macro and micro), toxins (synthetic preservatives, dyes, artificial sweeteners, heavy metals, etc.), and antinutrients they contain are incorporated into your cells and tissues. Since your body relies upon a steady stream of nutrients to function well, you should strive to give it the nutrients, not calories, it requires every day.

There are dozens to hundreds of different ways that you can eat, many of which have scientific validation to show they are the "best" diet for human health. An equally vast number of experts and influencers share different opinions on diet and nutrition, frequently directly contradicting one another. However, there is no one size fits all diet for every human being. It is illogical to believe this since there is so much biological and genetic diversity in humans. The best way to direct your diet is to have a genetic test (nutrigenomics) that can deliver personalized nutrition and fitness recommendations based on a saliva swab. These genetic tests can tell you whether your body processes carbohydrates, fats, and proteins efficiently, and what types of exercise your body will respond to best.

Nutrigenomics, or nutritional genomics, is the study of how your genes and nutrition interact. Variants in your genes help predict how your body will respond to nutrients, dietary components, and nutraceuticals. Moreover, it involves the study of how certain nutrients affect gene expression (epigenetics). Genes respond to environmental and dietary influences, particularly folate, choline, vitamins B2, B6, B12, and A, which help regulate gene expression. Armed with this knowledge, you can find out what nutrients turn your genes on or off, up or down. This exciting and developing field can evaluate dozens of genetic markers and determine risks associated with diet. For instance, nutrigenomics testing can help determine whether a person is likely to have an inflammatory reaction to saturated fat that could potentially increase cardiovascular disease risk. Variants on your FTO gene—a gene related to metabolism, energy expenditure, and body composition—reveals how well your body metabolizes fats and protein. Some of us have greater enzyme activity to convert beta-carotene to vitamin A, and this has to do with variants in BCO1 genes. Nutrigenomics permits an individual to adjust their nutrition to their personalized needs to reduce sweets cravings, diminish jitters caused by caffeine, lose weight or maintain a healthy weight, burn more fat with targeted exercise, and more.

During the average human's lifetime, more than 120,000 pounds of food will travel through the GI tract.[64] This is obviously a significant amount of food to process and represents a lot of opportunity for nutrients and dietary components to influence gene expression, gut health, immune health, and overall health. Your microbiome is particularly sensitive to dietary changes. Dietary alterations can trigger large, temporary shifts in the gut microbiome within twenty-four hours.[65] Absent a nutrigenomics test, you should focus on eating a balanced diet with as many fresh, whole foods as possible.

Eating fruits and vegetables provides fiber, which feeds probiotics, to build a healthy gut microbiome and protect gut health. Some prebiotic foods to consider include Jerusalem artichokes, mushrooms, steel-cut oats, chicory root, dandelion greens, garlic, onions, asparagus, barley, bananas, and apples. You should also eat probiotic foods daily. These include full-fat, low-sugar yogurt (in moderation), kimchi, kefir, coconut kefir, sauerkraut, fermented vegetables, kvass, apple cider vinegar, and pickles. Animal protein sources, like beef, chicken, and turkey, can also be consumed. Most research finds that eating meat does not negatively impact the gut microbiome, and those studies that do show a negative impact were in the context of a diet high in sugar or fat.[66,67] In fact, animal protein sources may have better effects on the gut microbiome than plant proteins because of their higher digestibility and the presence of antinutrients in plant proteins.[68] Whole grains may also have a beneficial effect on the gut microbiome,[69] but be careful with wheat (unless it's sprouted) because it may increase intestinal permeability, especially if it is laced with glyphosate—a widely used herbicide.[70,71] Glyphosate destroys your gut microbiome, reduces intestinal antioxidant capacity, and triggers intestinal inflammation.[72] Indeed, gluten sensitivities may be glyphosate sensitivities. Indeed, the same principles apply to eating for gut health as for overall health.

Just as important as choosing the right foods to include for gut health is, you should also avoid or limit certain foods. As mentioned earlier, wheat can be problematic if not sprouted. So too can other gluten-containing grain products such as barley, rye, bulgur, seitan, and triticale. This is because gluten (gliadin) increases zonulin production.[73] Zonulin is a group of proteins that regulates gut permeability at the cellular level.[74] The tight junctions in the intestines open wider when excess zonulin is produced, allowing macromolecules to escape the GI tract and trigger an inflammatory response. Left unchecked, this escape of macromolecules and consequential inflammatory response can dysregulate immune function leading to a host of autoimmune or autoinflammatory conditions.

Contrary to what the public has been sold for decades, highly refined industrial seed oils—canola, corn, soybean, cottonseed, safflower—are not heart healthy or otherwise beneficial to your health. Unlike traditional fats like butter, lard, olive oil, coconut oil, and ghee, the process to create these oils is anything but natural. First, seeds are heated to extreme temperatures, which oxidizes the unsaturated fatty acids, creating harmful byproducts. A petroleum-based solvent, frequently neurotoxic hexane, is used next to maximize oil extraction. Third, chemicals are used to deodorize the oils, forming trans fats. The last step of the process is to add more chemicals to improve the color of the oils. The result is a highly processed oil with lots of calories and very little nutrition that contains oxidized byproducts, chemical residues, and trans fats that all threaten human health. Additionally, higher PUFA (polyunsaturated fatty acids) oils like those mentioned are more prone to rancidity and oxidize even more when exposed to heat. While the effects of high-PUFA oils on gut permeability and the microbiome remain inconclusive, the fact that they can trigger an inflammatory response alone makes them worth limiting or avoiding.[75] Remember that PUFA levels in your body are also a key to ferroptosis activity.

Processed meats include any meat that has been altered to improve taste or extend its shelf life. This can be anything from salting to curing, smoking to fermenting, drying to canning, or the addition of chemical preservatives. Sausages, beef jerky, bacon, hot dogs, corned beef, and deli meats are all types of processed meat. Processed meat has consistently been linked to harmful health effects—high blood pressure, certain types of cancer, heart disease, and chronic obstructive pulmonary disease,[76,77,78,79,80] which is the result of a combination of the chemicals in the meat itself and the reality that people who eat a lot of processed meat tend to do other things that are not good for their health.

One of the problems with cured meats is the N-nitroso compounds they contain. These compounds are formed from nitrite (sodium nitrite), which is added as a preservative, flavor enhancer, and antimicrobial agent. Nitrosamines—compounds primarily formed when processed meats are exposed to high heat (above 266°F or 130°C)—are the most widely studied N-nitroso compounds. Some meats can be high in polycyclic aromatic hydrocarbons (PAHs) depending on how they are cooked. Smoking, grilling, barbecuing, and even roasting over an open fire can form PAHs, which are associated with cancer.[81] Processed meats sabotage gut health and can lead to chronic inflammation.[82]

Most baked and packaged goods are also ultra-processed and full of ingredients that are not beneficial to gut or human health. Artificial sweeteners, high fructose corn syrup, excess sugar and salt, synthetic preservatives, food dyes, surplus calories, emulsifiers (carboxymethylcellulose, polysorbate 80), and more lurk within these junk foods. Some of these ingredients have been associated with alterations in the gut microbiome and inflammation.[83,84] Moreover, processed foods often contain glycated proteins or lipids.[85] Advanced glycation end products (AGEs) are the final product of reactions where sugars spontaneously react with proteins (aminopeptides), fats (lipids), and nucleic acids. Amino-containing lipids are also subject to glycation and commonly a part of high-fat diets. A strong relationship with the accumulation of AGEs has been established with inflammaging (a chronic low-grade inflammation that can accelerate aging).[86] Oxidative stress increases as you age, which accelerates the shortening of telomeres (protective caps on the end of DNA strands and a marker for how youthful your cells are functioning), leading to cellular senescence and further exacerbating inflammation. Certain foods are more likely to produce AGEs when cooked, such as meat, seeds, margarine, mayonnaise, cheese, eggs, and nuts. Additionally, the way foods are cooked has a significant effect on their AGEs content. Deep frying, frying, roasting, grilling, broiling, and barbecuing each create these damaging molecules.

Consumption of AGEs from dietary sources increases both oxidation and inflammation, which can interfere with cell function and signaling. Left unchecked, the accumulation of AGEs leads to a host of health problems, including metabolic disorders (insulin resistance, diabetes), cancers, kidney disease, cardiovascular disease, neurodegenerative diseases, skin aging, and overall aging.[87] AGE is an appropriate acronym for these end products given their strong link to aging and harm to health.

Since the digestive tract is the first and principal site for the exposure to and absorption of AGEs, it is not surprising that they can negatively impact gut health. Indeed, scientists believe that the gut is one of the most susceptible organs to their negative effects,[88] which can have both local and systemic consequences. What the researchers have found is that AGEs increase intestinal permeability (leaky gut), contribute to dysbiosis, and alter enteric nervous system function and signaling.[89,90,91] AGEs represent a trifecta for disrupting gut and immune health.

It's cheap, convenient, and readily available, but fast food doesn't do your body any favors. The cornerstones of a diet geared towards a healthy gut microbiome provide fiber, probiotics, and a diversity of nutrient-dense foods. This is relatively nonexistant in fast food that is calorie-dense, lacks fiber, and contains loads of refined sugar, salt, and fat. A high-fat (the wrong fats) and high-calorie diet negatively alters gut permeability, inflammation, and affects your gut microbiome, tilting the microbes present towards obesity and chronic disease.[92,93,94,95,96] Trans fats (like partially hydrogenated oils), which are a man-made unsaturated fat abundant in fast foods, are known to contribute to dysbiosis, increase gut permeability, and amplify GI tract inflammation.[97] This may be why fried foods are associated with similar deleterious effects on the GI tract. Frying foods may deteriorate oils, increasing trans fats and the production of AGEs.[98] Overeating fast food can negatively impact both short- and long-term health, which is largely driven by disrupted metabolism, gut, and immune function.

Chronic or excess consumption of alcohol disturbs gut health and reduces the absorption of nutrients and water. Even single large alcohol binges can be harmful to the gut. Specifically, alcohol damages the intestinal mucosa, contributes to bacterial overgrowth, allows large molecules to escape the GI tract (increased intestinal permeability), facilitates the escape and relocation of toxins into the bloodstream, and promotes inflammation and tissue/organ damage.[99,100] Alcohol throws your gut out of balance, which triggers a cascade of events that dysregulates immune and metabolic homeostasis.

Whether dairy products can be consumed as part of a healthy diet or not is a controversial subject. Part of the problem with dairy is that it has been pasteurized since the mid-1900s and homogenized as well, which reduces its nutritional value and may make it less digestible in humans. Before this, all milk was consumed in its raw, natural, and unprocessed state. Pasteurization involves heating the milk to kill bacteria, yeasts, and molds, but it also destroys beneficial bacteria and enzymes. Homogenization applies extreme pressure to more evenly disperse the fatty acids in milk and improve its texture and taste. Interestingly, some research suggests that raw milk consumption reduces the risk of allergies and may reduce lactose intolerance.[101] Rapid heat treatments, like pasteurization, can alter the shape of milk proteins, flattening the molecules so their enzymes don't work.[102] While important to reduce foodborne infections, pasteurization is not completed without its costs.

Another issue is the presence of lactose (the primary milk sugar) and casomorphins (opioid peptides created when the primary protein in milk, casein, is digested). About 80 percent of cow's milk protein is casein. This protein breaks down in the stomach to produce casomorphins, which have similar structures to gliadin, suggesting consuming wheat and dairy (often done in modern Westernized diets) could trigger an amplified autoimmune and inflammatory response.[103] Therefore, dairy tears up the gut by causing dysbiosis, increased intestinal permeability, and may even act upon neurons in the enteric nervous system.

It is clear that many foods, or ingredients, have the potential to disrupt gut and immune function leading to an inflammatory response. Depending on your current diet and gut-immune health status, it can take from three to six months for dietary changes to be noticeable. If you have a strong intolerance or sensitivity to certain foods, you may notice improvements in a couple of weeks after eliminating the offending food. What you eat—and don't eat—has a significant impact on your gut, immune, and overall health.

Hydration

Water is essential for life! The average adult body is 50 to 65 percent water, 60 percent of which is inside your cells. Some organs, like the lungs, heart, and brain, are more than 70 percent water. It is necessary to lubricate joints, carry nutrients and oxygen to cells (your blood is more than 90 percent water), regulate body temperature, protect organs and tissues, absorb minerals and nutrients, flush out body waste, and reduce kidney burden. You lose water every day through urination, defecation, sweating, and breathing, making it vital that you hydrate daily.

The digestive system also depends on water. Water is involved in every step of the digestive process. It is a major component of saliva, which makes food easier to chew and swallow and contains enzymes that begin the breakdown of fats and carbohydrates. Watery juices in your stomach contain enzymes that break down proteins and carbohydrates. Water is also necessary to produce the protective mucosal lining of your stomach. As food moves through the GI tract, more watery secretions and enzymes are excreted into the small intestine, which aids the absorption of dietary components (amino acids, fatty acids, sugars). Most nutrient absorption occurs in the small intestine, and then these nutrients are transferred to the watery environment of your bloodstream. The large intestine also relies on water, leveraging it to dissolve soluble fiber and bulk with insoluble fiber to promote healthy bowel movements. There's no question that digestion would not occur efficiently without adequate water.

Drinking water comes from various origins, which may be subject to different treatments and contaminants. A combination of environmental conditions at the source, processing, storage, and distribution, produces distinct chemical, mineral, and microbial signatures of drinking water. The source of your drinking water dramatically shapes your gut microbiome.[104] Research shows that people who drink bottled and city water have divergent microbiomes when compared to people who drink well water. Moreover, people who drink less water have higher levels of *Campylobacter*—a group of bacteria associated with infections commonly called stomach flu—than those who drink higher amounts of water. Given how much water the average person should consume, drinking water and other beverages have a significant impact on gut-microbiome diversity.

Despite the popularity of the recommendation to drink eight glasses of water per day, most people need more than this to maintain optimum hydration levels. As a general guideline, the National Academies of Sciences, Engineering, and Medicine recommends that adult women get ninety-one ounces of fluid and adult men 125 ounces of fluid daily from both food and beverages.[105] Your kidneys have a remarkable capacity to flush out between 676 and 946 ounces of water every day, but they can only process about thirty-three ounces each hour. A more individualized approach to hydration, that considers water obtained from foods, is to drink half of your body weight in ounces each day. For instance, if you weigh 160 pounds, you should drink eighty ounces of water daily. This can be adjusted for physical activity level and hot climates as well.

Movement for Life

Most people understand that physical activity is important for physical health, some probably understand its importance for mood and mental health, but few likely realize how it affects gut health and immune function. Physical activity—any movement that burns energy—can involve walking, gardening, cycling, swimming, running, playing a sport, strength training, and a host of other activities that get your body moving. Keep in mind that your GI tract contains muscles (smooth muscle) as well, and when you move your skeletal muscles, you are also moving your digestive muscles to improve gut health.

More and more evidence is emerging to support a strong relationship between physical activity and gut–immune health. White blood cell levels increase temporarily during strenuous physical activity.[106] Depending on the intensity of the physical activity, the number of neutrophils circulating in your bloodstream and their activity changes. Moderate activity increases their activity, while strenuous activity decreases their activity.[107,108,109] The cytotoxic activity of natural killer cells and their levels also increases during and after brief intense exercise.[110] Contrarily, heavy prolonged exercise decreases natural killer cell activity.[111] Other research demonstrates that the movement of natural killer cells known to regulate immune responses, especially in autoimmune disease—CD56(bright) and CD16(-/dim)—increases after physical activity.[112] It is clear that physical activity has wide-ranging effects on immune function.

Specific to the effects of physical activity on autoimmunity, it does affect some of the immune cells involved in the development and progression of disease. T cells—helper CD4+ and cytotoxic CD8+—are an integral part of the adaptive immune system and play a role in the development of autoimmune disorders. CD4 cells can be further subdivided into Th1 (directs the fight against threats inside a cell, mainly viruses and bacteria that act like viruses), Th2 (regulates responses to threats outside cells, like bacteria, parasites, and toxins), Th17 (has overlap with Th1 cells, but primarily fights fungi), and Th22 (participates in mucosal defense, tissue repair, and wound healing) cells. Each type of T-helper cell has its own signals, called cytokines, that it sends to the rest of the immune system. Cytokines are inherently inflammatory and an imbalance in cytokine production by the various T-helper cells can signal the immune system to attack healthy cells. If one type of T-helper cell dominates signal sending (cytokine production), the other types of T-helper cell suppress their signaling efforts. Since Th1 cells specifically address intracellular threats, excess Th1 cytokine production can lead to organ-specific autoimmune attacks. When Th2 cell cytokine production is out of balance, allergies or systemic autoimmune attacks (e.g., lupus) can occur. Th17 cells play a little of both sides, but when they overproduce cytokines, it tends to look like a Th1 dominance situation. Th22 cells increase inflammation and tumor progression when overexpressed and can differentiate into Th1 or Th2 cells under certain conditions. Maintaining a balance in the activity of cytokine production of each one of these T-helper cell types decreases autoimmunity, promotes immune tolerance, and strengthens the ability of the immune system to fight infections. And the amount and diversity of microbes in your gut directly contributes to balanced immune function, substantially regulating immune cell development and homeostasis.

Your gut microflora substantially impacts your body functions through metabolic reprogramming (necessary for cell differentiation and proliferation and plays a role in immune balance), modifications in epigenetic expression, regulation of intestinal permeability (tight junctions), and the activation of specific receptors. Dysbiosis is characterized by a reduction in gut-microbiome diversity involving the loss of beneficial microbes (bacteroides and butyrate-producing bacteria) and a rise in pathogenic microbes. This shift in gut balance and diversity can activate an uncontrolled immune response that causes autoimmunity.[113] Furthermore, the amount of short-chain fatty acid butyrate produced by the gut microbiome affects the number and balance of T regulatory cells, which promote balanced immune function—the sweet spot where the immune system responds properly to harmful invaders but avoids attacking healthy body tissues and cells.[114] Dysbiosis deregulates intestinal permeability and initiates an inflammatory response that can result in autoimmunity in susceptible individuals. Bacteria found in the mucus layer of the intestines may hold the key to unlocking the mysterious interplay between autoimmunity and gut-microbiome health.

The cluster of microbes found in the human gastrointestinal tract plays protective, structural, and metabolic roles in intestinal function. One of the factors that influences microbial diversity and numbers is physical activity. Indeed, exercise can enhance the number of beneficial microbes, enhance microbial diversity, and help healthy bacteria thrive in the gut.[115] A higher abundance of health-promoting bacteria, including *Bifidobacterium* and *Akkermansia* (a bacteria important for metabolic health and the prevention of obesity), and greater microbial diversity has been observed in people who live an active lifestyle in comparison to their sedentary peers.[116,117,118] This enriched gut microbiome is associated with improved health and immune function.

Immune system function is also dependent on the byproducts of microbial metabolism—primarily acetate, propionate, and butyrate. Short-chain fatty acids are products of the bacterial fermentation of carbohydrates and proteins. All types of immune cells interact with these metabolites, which activate distinct signaling pathways.[119] Great attention is placed on butyrate since it is the major short-chain fatty acid affecting the immune system. A multitude of bacteria can produce butyrate, but the primary producers belong to the phylum Firmicutes (e.g., *Faecalibacterium parasitizes*, *Clostridium leptum*, *Eubacterium rectale*, and *Roseburia* spp.), while other phyla such as Actinobacteria, Bacterizes, Fusobacteria, Proteobacteria, Spirochaetes, and Hermitages can produce butyrate under certain conditions. Butyrate participates in the production of signaling molecules by GI cells, alters neutrophil and eosinophil activity, reduces inflammation, and strengthens intestinal tight junctions.[120] Physically fit individuals have higher levels of butyrate and short-chain fatty acids, and an increased abundance of key butyrate-producing bacteria, leading to improved gut health.[121] The good news is that both single-bouts and regular physical activity can even counter the activation of inflammatory pathways in people who are obese.[122] With the hormones the microbiome produces (e.g., GABA by *Lactobacilli* spp.; noradrenaline, dopamine, and serotonin by multiple bacterial species), the gut microbiome participates in endocrine system function. Its byproducts directly participate in gut-brain axis communication and butyrate and propionate serve as major energy sources for neurons and may even regulate the production of neurotransmitters by the central nervous system. All together ample evidence exists to show that immunity may chiefly be controlled by the gut.

Master Stress

Each of us experiences stress. We can't necessarily control how much stress we experience, but we can control our responses, develop greater coping strategies, and build up greater resilience to it. Stress begins in your brain when one of your senses, like sight, touch, or hearing, detects danger. Alarm signals are sent to the amygdala—an area of the brain primarily involved in emotional responses, memory, and decision-making, which interprets the messages from your senses. If danger is perceived (whether real or only perceived) it sends a distress signal to the main link between your nervous and endocrine systems, the hypothalamus. Downstream signals are sent that release hormones that alter physiological responses to respond to the danger. Once the danger has been avoided or neutralized, additional signals are sent to end the stress response and return physiological functions to normal. All of this happens so quickly you aren't even aware of it. While essential to avoid threats like an aggressive dog, it is less than ideal for you to be in a chronic stress response.

Chronic stress puts your health at risk as you are constantly bombarded with stress hormones that have the potential to disrupt virtually all your body's processes. Mental and emotional conditions like anxiety and depression can increase. You have a greater risk of heart disease, sleep problems, weight gain, muscle tension, and memory impairment. It even disrupts immune and digestive function.

Your mental, emotional, and physical health are not the only things that prolonged stress affects. It can also sabotage your intestinal barrier function and increase the uptake of potentially harmful molecules, like toxins, proinflammatory mediators, and antigens from the gut.[123] Altered gut microbiomes have also been observed during periods of psychological stress.[124] Long-term, stress may initiate immune reactions that increase the risk of chronic disease, including autoimmune and autoinflammatory conditions.

Don't Ignore Sleep

Sleep and digestion go together like tacos and Tuesdays. Digestive function can be diminished without restful sleep and poor digestion can lead to low-quality sleep. Your digestive system continues to work even while sleeping, although at a much slower rate. Gut tissues are also grown, repaired, and rebuilt during sleep, and the gut relies on glucose consumed during the day to fuel these processes. If you eat a large meal too close to bedtime, your digestive system will not have adequate time to rest and perform these vital processes.

Bacteria in the gut influence healthy sleep patterns by creating neurochemicals. In fact, microbe depletion can eliminate the production of serotonin and B6 in the gut, which directly influences sleep-wake cycles.[125] What this means is that your sleep cycle can shift to spend less time in non-REM sleep (including N3, which is the important restorative sleep stage) and more time in REM sleep. While the improved diversity in the gut microbiome is associated with better sleep, the presence of certain strains of bacteria is associated with poor sleep—*Lachnospiraceae*, *Corynebacterium*, and *Blautia*. So, sleep is not only dependent on the variety of microbes in your gut, but also on how many of certain phyla are present.[126] Knowing this may lead to the possibility of improving sleep quality by altering gut-microbiome composition.

With the intimate connection between the gut and nervous and immune function, it's no wonder that immune function is also closely related to sleep. Lack of or nonrestful sleep makes your immune system produce more proinflammatory cytokines, resulting in greater inflammation. Lack of sleep alters both innate and adaptive immune function, promoting a chronic and systemic inflammatory state and increasing the risk of various health disorders.[127]

A More Holistic Approach to Health Care

We need to shift away from seeking quick fixes to lifestyle diseases. The modern lifestyle has greatly contributed to disease burden as has the current medical paradigm of deploying rescue medicine—in the form of pills and surgery—to save us from poor lifestyle behaviors. This is even true of using herbs, dietary supplements, and essential oils to correct health conditions without addressing underlying lifestyle behaviors that contribute to the condition. Lifestyle adjustments can significantly improve responses to natural solutions.

YOUR HEALTH TREE

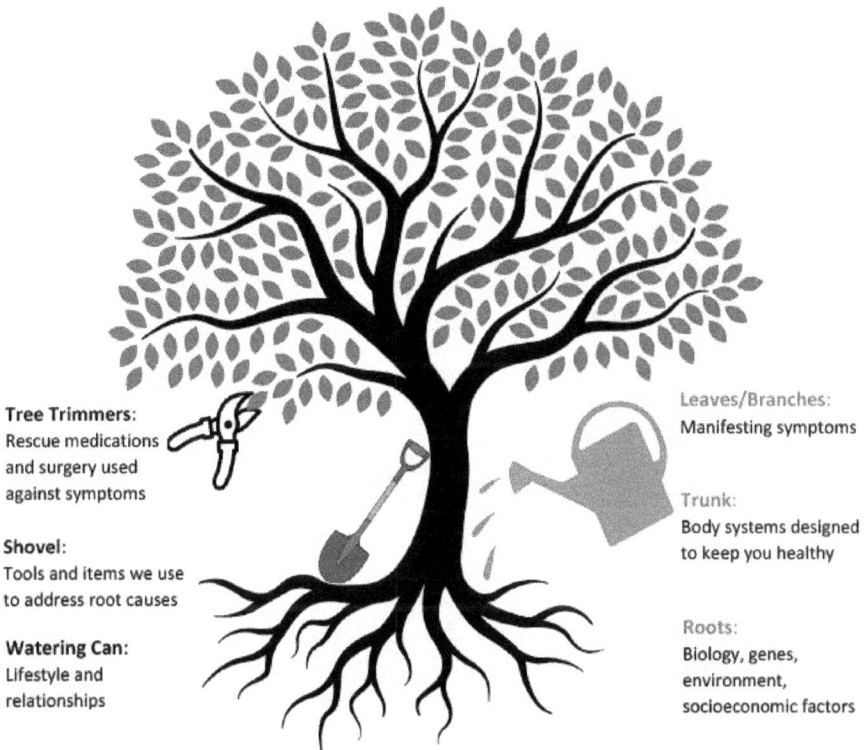

Tree Trimmers:
Rescue medications and surgery used against symptoms

Shovel:
Tools and items we use to address root causes

Watering Can:
Lifestyle and relationships

Leaves/Branches:
Manifesting symptoms

Trunk:
Body systems designed to keep you healthy

Roots:
Biology, genes, environment, socioeconomic factors

Roots: Genes predispose but do not predestine disease and illness. They require a trigger (lifestyle, environment) to manifest. The structure, function, growth, and distribution of your cells, tissues, and organs (biology) and environmental factors (exposure to chemicals, access to clean water, sanitation, etc.) also significantly influence risk. Socioeconomic factors, such as access to safe housing and proactive health care, are additional important factors.

Trunk: Your body is amazingly equipped with several key body systems to maintain a state of wellness.

Leaves/Branches: Manifesting symptoms are signs of corrective action that needs supported.

Watering Can: Lifestyle and relationship factors are the foundation of your health. These factors considerably affect whether your roots eventually develop illness/disease or health, making them the most important factors to focus on.

Shovel: Tools like herbs, dietary supplements, essential oils, massage, and physical therapy support your trunk (body systems) by aiding them to complete corrective action and by removing roadblocks that limit their activity and function.

Tree Trimmers: Rescue medicine (drugs, surgery) may thwart your body's corrective actions, causing your body to go to deeper levels to improve health. These tend to address things at a surface level and do not address the root cause.

4

HEALING THE GUT NATURALLY TO HEAL THE IMMUNE SYSTEM

Now that we've explored the connection between the gut and immunity, how can we heal the gut to heal the immune system? Healing the gut is nearly always the first step to reversing chronic health conditions involving dysregulated immune function. The root cause of an illness very likely involves your digestive system. Fortunately, healing the gut is a simple four-step process: 1) cleanse and reduce toxic burden, 2) strengthen gut-barrier integrity, 3) restore the gut microbiome, and 4) protect gut cells and tissues from further damage. Implementing this four-step process will improve gut health, immune health, and overall health.

Cleanse and Reduce Toxic Burden

The first step is intended to reduce the number of harmful microbes present in the GI tract. Dysbiosis, *Candida* overgrowth, small intestinal bacteria overload, and toxins can all damage cells in your intestinal wall. Damaged GI cells means more bacteria, toxins, and harmful molecules can escape the GI tract and enter the bloodstream. Moreover, your GI mucous membranes can be damaged, allowing bacteria biofilms— collections of bacteria that are protected by a layer of slime—to attach to the intestinal wall making them harder to eradicate. Imagine this like a rusty pipe. As the pipe rusts, holes open up inside that allow contents to leak out that shouldn't. At the same time, rust is establishing a home on the inside of the pipes. The goal of cleansing is to be selective in destroying harmful microbes while leaving healthy microbes largely intact—unlike antibiotics, which indiscriminately kill microbes (a scorched earth approach).

Before jumping in to proven gut-healing strategies, it's important to note that if your gut is unhealthy, it's likely to get worse before it gets better. Changing your gut microbiome alone can produce uncomfortable symptoms and even a Herxheimer reaction (also called a die-off, or Jarisch-Herxheimer reaction). This is a term used to describe a reaction during the clearance of pathogens (bacteria, fungi, viruses, yeasts, etc.) from the body with antimicrobials. It is believed to occur when endotoxins produced by massive numbers of dying pathogens overwhelm the body's ability to clear them out. This creates a toxic state that produces characteristic flu-like symptoms such as headache, fever, muscle aches, skin rashes, brain fog, and gastrointestinal problems (bloating, gas, diarrhea, and constipation). Die-off reactions usually occur when significant lifestyle changes are made: diet modification (switching from processed to whole foods—pathogens starve and die off rapidly), beginning probiotics (modifies the gut microbial balance to one with more good bacteria), or taking an antimicrobial substance (food, herb, supplement, or drug). This type of reaction will usually occur hours (1–2) to days (up to 10) after the lifestyle modification is implemented.

The risk of die-off reactions may be reduced by backing off on the amount of the antimicrobial substance consumed, making a dietary change more gradually, or reducing the dosage of probiotics taken. In addition, a digestive enzyme (especially one with bromelain and proteases) may reduce reactions to new foods added to the diet by facilitating better absorption of proteins and nutrients new to your body.

Cleansing should start with the colon because if this elimination channel is plugged up, cleansing other areas of the body will likely just create a logjam of toxins and dead microbes in the colon. Frankly, the GI tract must be unclogged before it can be cleansed of pathogens and toxins.

Colon cleanses involve bulking the stool (high-fiber products) and stimulating the GI tract to move this waste out of the colon efficiently. A third option is enemas or colonics, which work a little faster than herbs. Herbs affect the GI tract in different ways and subsequently produce different results. Pick the way you want to cleanse the bowel, gentle long game (fibers) or more rapid (stimulant herbal laxatives), or quickly (enema, colonic), and go for it, then continue the cleansing process by focusing on pathogenic microbe reduction.

Fiber

One of the gentlest ways to move the bowel is to take fiber supplements. Fiber is basically the parts of plant foods that your body doesn't digest and absorb. It is classified into two types: soluble and insoluble. Soluble fiber dissolves in water to form a gel-like material and consists of pectin and gums. Insoluble fiber doesn't dissolve in water and includes cellulose and hemicellulose. They each have unique benefits, which extend beyond promoting bowel regularity and health. In general, fiber supplements are considered safe to take daily, but in rare cases you could develop a dependence on the fiber to have a bowel movement.

Soluble fiber dissolves and ferments in your gut, providing nutrients for your gut microbiome. It can also improve blood sugar and cholesterol levels. It does so by slowing and reducing their absorption.[128] Foods with soluble fiber include apples, blueberries, lentils, beans, nuts, oatmeal, and chia seeds.

Insoluble fiber attracts water into your stool, which makes it softer and easier to pass. By doing so, it can help reduce the risk of hemorrhoids and promote bowel regularity. It also may promote weight loss and reduce the risk of colorectal cancer.[129,130] Foods with insoluble fiber include pears, apples, seeds, walnuts, almonds, and kale.

Psyllium contains high levels of soluble fiber and is commonly used as a bulk laxative.[131] When psyllium seed husk is mixed with water, it forms into a gel-like substance that helps ease stool from the bowels.[132]

Typical dosage: 3–24 grams; follow supplement label instructions

Cautions/Contraindications: Choking may occur if not taken with sufficient water (at least eight ounces), fecal impaction, GI tract narrowing, bowel obstruction, swallowing disorders, colorectal cancer, antipsychotics, anticonvulsants, lithium, metformin

Potential adverse effects: Generally well tolerated, abdominal discomfort, changes in bowel movement, stomach upset, flatulence, nausea

Containing both insoluble and soluble fiber, fatty acids, protein, and phytoestrogens, flaxseed is a bulk-forming laxative that helps relieve constipation. Its insoluble fibers include cellulose and lignan, whereas its soluble fibers consist of mucilage gums. Interestingly, preclinical research suggests that flaxseed oil and mucilage are helpful for both diarrhea and constipation.[133]

Typical dosage: 10–25 grams, twice daily; follow supplement label instructions

Cautions/Contraindications: Medications for high blood pressure and diabetes, antibiotics, blood-thinning drugs

Potential adverse effects: Generally well tolerated, bloating, diarrhea, stomachache

A tried-and-true remedy for constipation with decades of use, prune juice (dried plum juice) has traditionally been used for a variety of ailments including high blood pressure, fever, and jaundice. Eating prunes or drinking prune juice provides insoluble and soluble fiber, which mobilizes the digestive system. Remarkably eating just ten prunes provides nearly a quarter of the recommended daily fiber for adults. It contains high levels of the known laxative sorbitol—a sugar alcohol that ferments in the gut and draws water into stool. Dried prunes contain higher levels of sorbitol than prune juice. Taking it consistently softens the stool and increases the frequency of bowel movements. It is noteworthy that some people find that prune juice is more effective than psyllium.

Typical dosage: 55–200 grams (about 1/4 to 1 cup) of 100 percent juice daily; 80–120 grams of whole prunes (about 8 to 12 prunes) daily

Cautions/Contraindications: Ulcerative colitis, irritable bowel syndrome, kidney disease, diabetes, blood-thinning drugs

Potential adverse effects: Generally well tolerated, bloating, flatulence, dark stools

Stimulant Herbal Laxatives

Stimulant laxatives work by speeding up peristalsis—the involuntary rhythmic contraction and relaxation of GI tract muscles to propel food and fluids through your digestive tract—and accelerating the transit of food and liquids through the GI tract. These are most commonly used short-term—one to two weeks—but some people find that a single use can be very cleansing. Herbal laxatives contain anthranoids that stimulate cells in the intestines to keep things moving. They also reduce fluid absorption from the intestines into the body and enhance fluid secretion in the colon, resulting in softer stools. Two of the most popular stimulant herbal laxatives are cascara sagrada and senna leaf.

Found in some commercial laxative products, senna leaf is approved by the US FDA as an over-the-counter category III digestive aid.[134] Its safety and efficacy for occasional constipation have been proven in clinical research.[135] The active compounds in senna are anthraquinones (emodin and rhein) and dianthrone glycosides (sennoside A and B), which are known to have laxative effects.[136] Anthraquinones trigger an irritation response in the colon that causes colon contractions, helping facilitate regular bowel movements. Sennosides A and B reach the large intestine without undergoing changes and then are metabolized by bacteria into active metabolites (rhein and thein-anthrone). As mentioned, senna also reduces reabsorption of water and electrolytes in the colon, which leaves more water in the colon to soften the stool. Senna usually takes about eight hours to produce results, so it is often taken at bedtime to allow it to work overnight. For bowel-cleansing purposes, senna should be used for a few days, but no longer than one week.

Typical dosage: Adults—Dose providing 17.2 mg sennosides, once or twice daily; Adolescents/Teens (12–17)—17.2 mg sennosides daily;

Children (6–11)—8.6 mg sennosides daily; Children (2–5)—4.3 mg sennosides daily; follow supplement label instructions because of great variance in type and strength of preparations

Cautions/Contraindications: Not for long-term use to avoid bowel dependence, limit use to one week, GI pain of unknown origin, bowel obstruction, diarrhea, acute intestinal inflammation, digoxin, warfarin

Potential adverse effects: Generally well tolerated when used short-term at appropriate doses, stomach discomfort or cramps, diarrhea, flatulence, nausea or vomiting, bloating, urine discoloration, fecal urgency, reversible colon discoloration

Once approved as on over-the-counter laxative (FDA approval was removed because of insufficient evidence of efficacy, not safety), cascara sagrada bark has been used as a medicine for decades. Cascara sagrada also contains anthraquinone glycosides (primarily cascarosides A, B, C, and D), but it is milder than senna in its action. It needs to contain a minimum of 7 percent cascarosides to be effective. Like senna, cascara sagrada should only be used for a few days for bowel-cleansing purposes, but no more than one week.

Typical dosage: Follow supplement label instructions

Cautions/Contraindications: Not for long-term use to avoid bowel dependence, limit use to one week, bowel obstruction, acute intestinal inflammation, Crohn's disease, ulcerative colitis, appendicitis, stomach ulcers, abdominal pain of unknown origin, digoxin, warfarin

Potential adverse effects: Generally well tolerated when used short-term, mild abdominal discomfort, stomach cramps

Colonics and Enemas

Other bowel-cleansing options include colonics and enemas. The basic principle behind colonics (colon hydrotherapy) and enemas is the same, to flush out leftover waste from the colon by introducing water into the rectum. The primary difference between the two procedures is the methods used. Enemas are more a short-cut or quick approach where water—usually from eight to thirty-two ounces—is inserted through the rectum via a tube and held for up to twenty minutes before expelling.

The water travels about six to eight inches into the colon, meaning it is primarily cleansing the sigmoid colon (the lower part of the colon). Contrarily, colonics involve large amounts of water (330 to 1,690 ounces), two tubes, and a proctoscope that slowly saturates your entire colon with water. One tube inserts the water while the second tube carries water and waste matter out of the body. Because of this, colonics tend to be more soothing and promote more complete cleansing. While enemas can be self-administered and performed at home, colonics are performed by a health-care professional (colon therapist). The goal of both is to remove waste from the colon, improve digestion, and prevent constipation.

Antimicrobials

Once you have cleansed your colon using your preferred method, it is time to move onto the next stage of cleansing: antimicrobial agents. This effort focuses largely on reducing counts of harmful (pathogenic) bacteria and yeast in the GI tract, leveraging essential oils, herbs, and phages. This is usually through short-term use of these antimicrobial solutions—ten to fourteen days (see following table).

When it comes to antimicrobial activity, it's hard to beat essential oils. Many of them have demonstrated broad-spectrum antimicrobial activity against some of the most common pathogens that inhabit the GI tract. And, more importantly, they are not associated with pathogen resistance due to natural variations in their chemical composition. As you can see in the below table, the greatest effects will be obtained by using a blend of essential oils to target the most pathogen species. While dozens of essential oils could be used to reduce pathogen load in the digestive system, clove, lemongrass, oregano, peppermint, thyme have been selected because of their activity against the main target pathogens.

Herbs also have antimicrobial properties, but they are generally gentler and milder in nature than their essential oil cousins. Popular herbs to use for cleansing and digestive support include garlic, ginger, and usnea (a secondary metabolite of lichens rich in usnic acid and polyphenols). If parasites are a concern, black walnut is a frequent herb of choice. If you choose the herbal route, you may want to rotate through the list of herbs, using one for seven to ten days at a time, then resting a few days before starting the next herb.

Another emerging option to combat certain bacteria are phages—viruses that infect and replicate only in bacterial cells. Also called bacteriophages or cobiotics, these microbes are very species-specific and typically only infect a single bacterial species, or even specific strains within a species of bacteria. Once attached to a bacterial cell, phages hijack the bacteria's internal cellular structures to reproduce phage proteins, inhibiting or destroying the bacteria. Many phages target *E. coli*, making them good options for a very common pathogen in the GI tract. Like essential oils, a cocktail of phages targeting multiple bacteria will be most efficient in your cleansing regimen.

Common Infections of the GI Tract and Natural Antimicrobials to Combat Them

Infection	Pathogen	Symptoms	Transmission	Diagnosis	Antimicrobial Solution
"Food poisoning" B. cereus infection	*Bacillus cereus*	Nausea, vomiting, abdominal cramps, diarrhea	Ingestion of contaminated fish, dairy, meat, cereals, sauces, soups, rice, and veggies	Testing of food eaten and/or stool/vomit for presence of *B. cereus*	Clove EO, oregano EO, Peppermint EO, Thyme EO; ginger, usnea; bacteriophage PBC1
Campylobacteriosis "stomach flu"	*Campylobacter jejuni*	Fever, diarrhea, headache, nausea or vomiting, stomach cramps; sometimes dysentery, autoimmune conditions, or organ damage	Eating undercooked or uncooked food (chicken, produce, seafood), raw dairy products, untreated water	Testing of stool for presence of *C. jejuni*; extreme cases may require a blood test	Clove EO, oregano EO, peppermint EO, thyme EO; garlic; type III phages NCTC 12672, 12673, 12674, and 12678
Cholera	*Vibrio cholerae*	Diarrhea (very watery), intense thirst,	Consumption of contaminated food or water	Testing of stool for presence	Oregano EO (carvacrol); garlic, ginger

		muscle cramps, poor urine output, restlessness, weakness, vomiting; sometimes kidney failure		of *V. cholerae*, or rectal swab	(6-gingerol); bacteriophage ICP1
C. diff infection	*Clostridioides difficile*	Persistent abdominal pain, watery diarrhea, swollen or distended abdomen, fever, rapid heart rate, loss of appetite; severe cases may cause septicemia or bowel perforation	Conditions that compromise gut immunity (e.g., overgrowth of *C. diff* after antibiotic use, inflammatory bowel disease, immunosuppression), health-care-acquired infection	Testing of stool for toxins *C. diff* produces, blood test, or imaging	Oregano EO, thyme EO; cinnamon bark EO is most active; bacteriophages phiCD119, phiC2, phiCD27, phiCD6356, phiCD38-2, phiMMP02, phiMMP04, phi CDHM1
"Food poisoning" **C. perfringens** **infection** **gastroenteritis**	*Clostridium perfringens*	Mild stomach cramps, watery diarrhea; does not usually include fever or vomiting	Eating contaminated meat or poultry that has been left out too long or is undercooked	Usually based on symptoms, stool sample testing for *C. perfringens*	Thyme EO; sandalwood EO is highly active; garlic, ginger; bacteriophage CPs2
E. coli infection	*Escherichia coli*	Watery diarrhea, dysentery, abdominal cramps, low fever, chills, general malaise, fatigue, loss of appetite, nausea or vomiting; complications may include hemolytic uremic syndrome	Ingestion of contaminated food or water, poor handwashing	Testing of stool for presence of Shiga toxin-producing *E. coli* (STEC)	Clove EO, lemongrass EO, oregano EO, peppermint EO, thyme EO; garlic, ginger; *Escherichia* virus T1-7 (phages), *Escherichia* virus M13 (phage), *Escherichia* virus Lambda (phage)

H. pylori infection	Helicobacter pylori	Dull or burning stomach pain, unplanned weight loss, bloating, loss of appetite, nausea and vomiting (possibly bloody), indigestion, dark stools (blood in the stool); complications include stomach ulcer and stomach cancer	Kissing, poor handwashing, and possibly contaminated water and wood	Breath test, stool test, upper endoscopy	Clove EO, lemongrass EO, oregano EO, peppermint EO, thyme EO; garlic, ginger; bacteriophage 1961P, De-M53-M, Fr-B41-M, HP1, KHP30, phiHp33, pt-1293-U, sw-577-G
Candidiasis	Candida albicans, C. auris	White, yellow, or brown mucus or string-like substance in stool, froth or foam in stool, diarrhea, headache, fatigue, flatulence, cravings for sweets, skin itching	Antibiotic use, inflammatory bowel disease, ulcerative colitis, Crohn's disease, compromised immune function, unmanaged diabetes, oral contraceptives use, smoking, stress, excess alcohol consumption, corticosteroids use, excess consumption of refined carbs, yeast, or sugar	Stool test, culture swab, endoscopy	C. albicans: Clove EO, lemongrass EO, oregano EO, peppermint EO, thyme EO; garlic, ginger, usnea

C. auris: Clove EO; cinnamon bark is also highly active |

Antimicrobial essential oils (clove, lemongrass, oregano, peppermint, and thyme)

Typical dosage: Add 1 drop of each oil to a "0" size capsule, fill the rest with carrier oil (MCT, olive, black cumin seed, or avocado oil), and take morning and evening with a meal

Cautions/Contraindications: Pregnancy, lactation, iron-deficiency anemia, MAOI antidepressants, blood-thinning drugs,

antibiotics/antifungals, anticholinergic/cholinergic drugs, diabetes drugs, barbiturates, cyclosporine, caffeine
Potential adverse effects: Generally well tolerated orally, burp back (eructation), abdominal pain, nausea, vomiting, diarrhea

Herbs (garlic, ginger, usnea, and black walnut)

Typical dosage: Aged garlic, 400–500 mg, twice daily, with meals
Cautions/Contraindications: Bleeding conditions, prior to surgery, blood-thinning drugs, blood pressures meds, diabetes drugs, protease inhibitors, antiretroviral drugs
Potential adverse effects: Generally well tolerated orally, body odor, bad breath, abdominal pain, flatulence, nausea

Typical dosage: Ginger, 500–1000 mg, twice daily, with meals
Cautions/Contraindications: Bleeding conditions, heart conditions, prior to surgery, blood-thinning drugs, blood pressure meds
Potential adverse effects: Generally well tolerated orally, abdominal discomfort, burping, heartburn, diarrhea, throat irritation

Typical dosage: Usnea tincture, as instructed on the supplement label
Cautions/Contraindications: Pregnancy, lactation, liver disease or failure, not for long-term use (10 days maximum)
Potential adverse effects: GI issues, nausea, diarrhea, weakness or fatigue

Typical dosage: Green (unripe) black walnut tincture, as instructed on the product label, between meals (best timing is first thing in the morning, then again before lunch and dinner)
Cautions/Contraindications: Pregnancy, lactation, not for long-term use (10 days maximum), tree nut allergy
Potential adverse effects: generally well tolerated orally, GI upset

Phages

Typical dosage: Phage blend, as instructed on the product label
Cautions/Contraindications: None currently known
Potential adverse effects: Generally well tolerated

Heavy Metal Detoxification

Heavy metals—lead, mercury, cadmium, and arsenic—detoxification is an optional but valuable part of cleansing. We are exposed to and accumulate heavy metals from foods, water, the ground we walk on, products we use, cigarettes, pesticides, herbicides, insecticides, paints, batteries, construction materials, plumbing pipes, and even certain medications. Heavy metals bind to parts of your cells that prevent organs from functioning well. When it comes to heavy metal detoxification, you need solutions that mobilize (remove them from tissues they are stored in) and chelate (bind to and shuttle them to excretory channels) them for removal, as well as something like glutathione to facilitate elimination.

Three good options for heavy metals are nature's chelators, cilantro and chlorella, and oral glutathione. Cilantro and chlorella are a one-two combination for the removal of heavy metals that should be used together. Cilantro mobilizes more toxins than it can carry out of the body, meaning that without a companion like chlorella, you could simply relocate heavy metals from safer areas of storage in the body (like fat tissue) to more vital tissue like nervous or muscular tissue. Chlorella has excellent binding capacity and helps pick up the slack for cilantro. Together, they help facilitate the removal of heavy metals from cells and tissues, allowing them to function more efficiently.

Typical dosage: Alcohol-free cilantro tincture, as instructed on the product label
Cautions/Contraindications: Bleeding disorders, prior to surgery, blood-thinning drugs, photosensitizing drugs
Potential adverse effects: Diarrhea, stomachache

Typical dosage: Alcohol-free chlorella tincture, as instructed on the product label
Cautions/Contraindications: Mold sensitivity (cross-allergenicity), iodine sensitivity, immunodeficiency, blood-thinning drugs, photosensitizing drugs
Potential adverse effects: Generally well tolerated orally, abdominal cramps, constipation, diarrhea, fatigue, nausea, photosensitivity, stool discoloration

As mentioned earlier, glutathione is a major antioxidant inside cells. It is also considered your body's master detoxifier since it tirelessly works to eliminate heavy metals, mycotoxins, harmful chemicals (e.g., parabens, phthalates), and hundreds of other toxic substances lurking inside your body. Glutathione binds to these toxins so they can safely and effectively be eliminated from your body.[137] By doing so, glutathione reduces the risk of renal, cardiovascular, musculoskeletal, and neurological conditions. Although you do produce glutathione in the liver, today's toxic world full of chemicals and modern lifestyles often makes it necessary to boost it through supplementation.

Typical dosage: S-Acetyl L-Glutathione, 100–300 mg, daily
Cautions/Contraindications: None currently known
Potential adverse effects: Generally well tolerated orally

Liver and Kidneys Support

Next, you should support your detoxification and elimination organs, specifically the liver and kidneys. The liver is the primary organ in your body that helps metabolize and eliminate toxins. Its primary function is to filter and process blood that passes through the digestive tract. A liver detox can be performed in several different ways and often includes colon cleansing, which you should have already completed. Some choose to drink only vegetable and fruit juices, while others take herbs that aid liver function and the processing of toxins. Common herbs used to support healthy liver function include milk thistle (silymarin), dandelion root, turmeric, and artichoke leaf, and these are often found combined in liver-supporting supplements.

Note: Typical doses listed below are for taking each of the herbs individually. Amounts in a combination supplement may be lower.

Containing two powerful antioxidants—silymarin and silibinin, milk thistle has been used for liver support for hundreds of years. Your first line of defense against free radicals are the antioxidant enzymes superoxide dismutase (SOD), glutathione peroxidase (GSH-Px), and catalase that help remove precursors to free radical production. Metal-binding proteins—transferrin, lactoferrin, haptoglobin, hemopexin, metallothionein, ceruloplasmin, ferritin, albumin, myoglobin, and so on—also participate in your front-line defenses. Unfortunately, this level of free radical defense is not foolproof and some radicals do bypass this level, which can lead to cellular and tissue damage. The second line of defense deals with fully formed free radicals and includes glutathione (GSH) and thioredoxin systems. Milk thistle partly supports liver function by acting as a free radical scavenger (antioxidant) itself and activating the aforementioned defenses.[138]

Typical dosage: Milk thistle (standardized to 70%+ silymarin) 140 mg, three times daily; or 250–760 mg, once daily

Cautions/Contraindications: Allergy to Asteraceae (Compositae) family, diabetes drugs, ledipasvir, sofosbuvir, morphine, raloxifene, sirolimus, tamoxifen, blood-thinning drugs

Potential adverse effects: Generally well tolerated orally, bloating, diarrhea, heartburn, flatulence, nausea

Traditionally used as a liver tonic (exerts a restorative, cleansing, and protective effect on the liver), dandelion root also possesses antioxidant properties. It is a digestive bitter, which are substances that stimulate the production of bile and enhance bile flow from the liver. Bile is a complex fluid secreted by your liver and stored in your gallbladder that is critical for the absorption of fats and is also involved in protein and starch metabolism. Healthy bile production and storage is intricately connected to healthy liver function and detoxification because it carries all kinds of waste products, including toxins, to be eliminated from the body.

Typical dosage: 500–1,575 mg daily, with 8–12 ounces of water

Cautions/Contraindications: Bleeding disorders, allergy to Asteraceae (Compositae) family, prior to surgery, renal impairment, diabetes drugs, blood-thinning drugs, lithium, potassium-sparing diuretics, quinolone antibiotics

Potential adverse effects: Generally well tolerated orally, diarrhea, heartburn, stomachache

Turmeric is primarily known for its anti-inflammatory activity, but it also has antioxidant properties and has been used to protect the liver against oxidative stress. Clinical research shows that curcumin, the major polyphenol in turmeric herb, favorably affects liver function and helps reduce the accumulation of fats in the liver.[139] Turmeric's active compounds also enhance the activity of pathways involved in detoxification.[140,141] Turmeric is liver protective and supportive, and therefore strengthens your liver's detoxification processes.

Typical dosage: Standardized turmeric, 500 mg, twice daily; full-spectrum turmeric, 450–700 mg, twice daily

Cautions/Contraindications: HLA-B35 gene (higher risk of liver injury), bile duct obstruction, gallstones, bleeding disorders, infertility, prior to surgery, chemotherapy drugs, calcium channel blockers, beta-blockers, blood-thinning drugs, diabetes drugs, sulfasalazine, immunosuppressive meds, topoisomerase inhibitors

Potential adverse effects: Generally well tolerated orally, heartburn, GERD, diarrhea, bloating, nausea, vomiting

Like dandelion root, artichoke leaf is a digestive bitter and provides antioxidant protection to support liver health and bile flow. It contains the powerful antioxidant polyphenols luteolin and chlorogenic acid. Dandelion root augments enzymes and pathways involved in detoxification and disease progression.[142] It also boosts antioxidant levels and activity in the liver, including SOD, to help protect the liver against oxidative stress and liver injury.[143] Overall, artichoke leaf extract is an important herb for liver support and restoration.

Typical dosage: 320–640 mg, three times daily

Cautions/Contraindications: Pregnancy, lactation, bile duct obstruction, allergy to Asteraceae (Compositae) family, gallstones, diabetes drugs, high blood pressure meds

Potential adverse effects: Generally well tolerated orally, diarrhea, abdominal pain, hunger, flatulence, nausea

Your kidneys remove wastes—including toxins—and extra fluid form the body in the form of urine. They filter about half a cup of blood every minute to do so. They also remove acid produced by cells and help maintain a healthy balance of water, minerals, and salts in your blood. Each kidney contains about a million filtering units called nephrons, which work in two stages. The glomerulus in your nephrons filter the blood and the tubules remove waste and return necessary substances back to the blood. If you experience water retention, have high blood pressure (a sign of sodium retention in the kidneys), or have unusual fatigue, your kidneys may be calling out for a little assistance.

There are several ways to help your kidneys filter better. First and foremost, you should drink plenty of water as mentioned in the lifestyle chapter. Certain foods are also kidney supportive including lemons, oranges, carrots, bananas, parsley, cilantro, celery, apples, and strawberries. There are also herbs that are frequently used to aid the kidneys in their responsibilities to remove waste and excess water: uva ursi and dandelion root (with as a bonus that it supports the liver as well). For best results, these herbs are frequently combined into one supplement, often at lower amounts than what they would be used at as a single herb.

Uva ursi, also called bearberry, because bears eat the fruit, has been used medicinally for centuries. It contains several active compounds, including arbutin, hydroquinone, and tannins that reduce inflammation, fight infection, and influence mucous membranes. Uva ursi is commonly used for urinary tract infections (UTIs) because of its antimicrobial and antiadhesive—interferes with microbe adhesion to cells in the urinary tract, thereby protecting against UTIs—activity.[144] It is believed to be most effective if your urine is more alkaline than acidic. It is also considered a diuretic (substance that increases the production of urine) and kidney tonic.

Typical dosage: Uva ursi standardized to 20 percent arbutins, as instructed on the product label for up to one week

Cautions/Contraindications: Pregnancy, lactation, children under 12, not for long-term use (limit use to one week), kidney disease, retinal thinning, P-glycoprotein substrate drugs (apixaban, colchicine,

cyclosporine, dabigatran, digoxin, edoxaban, rivaroxaban, and tacrolimus), urinary acidifying agents
Potential adverse effects: Generally well tolerated, nausea, vomiting, stomach upset, diarrhea

Dandelion root is also a diuretic, so it helps promote waste removal in the urine.[145] The tea is often used for a kidney cleanse. Remarkably, dandelion root extract prevented kidney and liver damage caused by paracetamol and in preclinical models.[146,147] Dandelion is an excellent detoxifying herb because of its effects on both the kidneys and liver.

Typical dosage: 500–1,575 mg daily, with 8–12 ounces of water; or one cup of dandelion root tea daily
Cautions/Contraindications: Bleeding disorders, allergy to Asteraceae (Compositae) family, prior to surgery, renal impairment, diabetes drugs, blood-thinning drugs, lithium, potassium-sparing diuretics, quinolone antibiotics
Potential adverse effects: Generally well tolerated orally, diarrhea, heartburn, stomachache

Avoid Nonessential Antibiotic and Synthetic Drugs Use

More than seventy years of antibiotics use fighting infectious illnesses, and their widespread overuse, has led to reduced effectiveness. Additionally, we now have a clear understanding of how these antimicrobial agents affect gut health. Antibiotics are well known to have a negative impact on microbiome diversity and function, which can have a negative impact on humans.[148] In fact, even a single antibiotic treatment in healthy individuals contributes to long-lasting detrimental shifts in the gut microbiome.[149] Not to mention their contribution to the development of superbugs resistant to antimicrobial drugs. That's why it's important to only use antibiotics when absolutely necessary.

To add to the negative effects of antibiotics on the gut, they also disrupt intestinal barrier function, further increasing inflammation.[150] In other words, antibiotics make your intestinal barrier function less stable, which allows molecules to escape into the bloodstream that can trigger a reaction. Emerging research even suggests that antibiotics interfere with enteric nervous system function.[151] Specifically, antibiotics alter neurocircuitry and neurochemical production in the gut. In essence, antibiotics cross wires and hinder production signaling pathways and molecules so your second brain is disorganized and clumsy.

Another class of drugs that is known to wreak havoc on gut health is non-steroidal anti-inflammatory drugs (NSAID). Popped like candy in modern times, NSAIDs reduce pain, inflammation, and fever, and help prevent blood clots. If overused, NSAIDs can cause great harm and are one of the leading causes of hospitalization among people admitted to hospitals for medication side effects. They are also prone to causing GI injuries. NSAID drugs can increase leaky gut syndrome up to threefold after only one to seven days of use.[152,153] Moreover, NSAIDs can adversely affect the gut microbiome.[154,155] It is ironic that an anti-inflammatory drug can actually cause intestinal inflammation and contribute to factors that could make the inflammatory cascade worse over time.

We are also beginning to learn that many common medications also affect the gut microbiome.[156,157] Both positive and negative effects have been identified. Interestingly, the diabetes drug metformin encourages the growth of short-chain fatty acids, which reduces drug efficacy and helps explain part of its therapeutic function, as well as some side effects—diarrhea, bloating, and nausea.[158] And this is just one example of gut-microbiome effects that drugs have. Moreover, your gut-microbiome diversity can affect the efficacy and safety of drugs by augmenting bioavailability and transforming drug actives into metabolites.[159] A greater understanding or how medications influence gut-microbiome diversity and function, and medication efficacy and side effects will help unlock the possibility to better individualize condition treatments. What we know now is that your gut microbiome reflects a combination of lifestyle factors and medications used.

Body Odor while Cleansing

Occasionally, people experience a strong body odor when cleansing and detoxifying. Accumulated waste and toxins are not only evacuated from the body in the feces and urine but also released from sweat glands. Stimulating your elimination channels, especially if you have a high toxic load, can cause a foul body odor. It's similar to why the skin of alcoholics, or people who drink a lot of alcohol, smells like alcohol. Your body considers alcohol a toxin and excretes it through your pores or sweat glands.

Sweat itself doesn't smell, but when it mixes with bacteria on your skin, it has a distinct odor. While your armpit microbiome consists of varies bacterial species, it is dominated by *Corynebacterium* and *Staphylococcus* species, which are key contributors to body odor, along with *Cutibacterium*. These microbes break down molecules secreted from your sweat glands and release malodorous byproducts. Fortunately, essential oils inhibit these odor-causing bacteria.

To combat armpit odor during cleansing, mix the following in a 4-ounce squeeze container (preferably HDPE No. 2 or PET plastic):

2 ounces of distilled water
1.5 ounces of apple cider vinegar
4 drops rosemary essential oil
3 drops eucalyptus essential oil
3 drops of tea tree essential oil
2 drops arborvitae essential oil

Shake well before each use. Add several drops of the blend to a clean cotton ball and cleanse your armpits, twice daily.

Targeted Supplementation to Replenish, Strengthen, Restore, and Protect

Once you've made it past cleansing, it is time to focus on replenishing (repopulating) your gut microbiome, strengthening intestinal barrier function, restoring damaged tissues, and protecting GI cells and tissues from further damage by limiting ferroptosis. People with DNA methylation issues or certain genetic mutations will also need to aid DNA methylation as part of the process. Fortunately, all of this can be done simultaneously, rather than in stages. Indeed, the gut microbiome significantly influences tight junctions (intestinal barrier function), so it is important to perform these tasks at the same time. Supplements that balance ferroptosis will also be explored since this is closely related to immune health, particularly disrupted immune function, and at least partly regulated by the gut microbiome. With patience, consistency, and high-quality supplements, you can heal your gut and therefore your immune system.

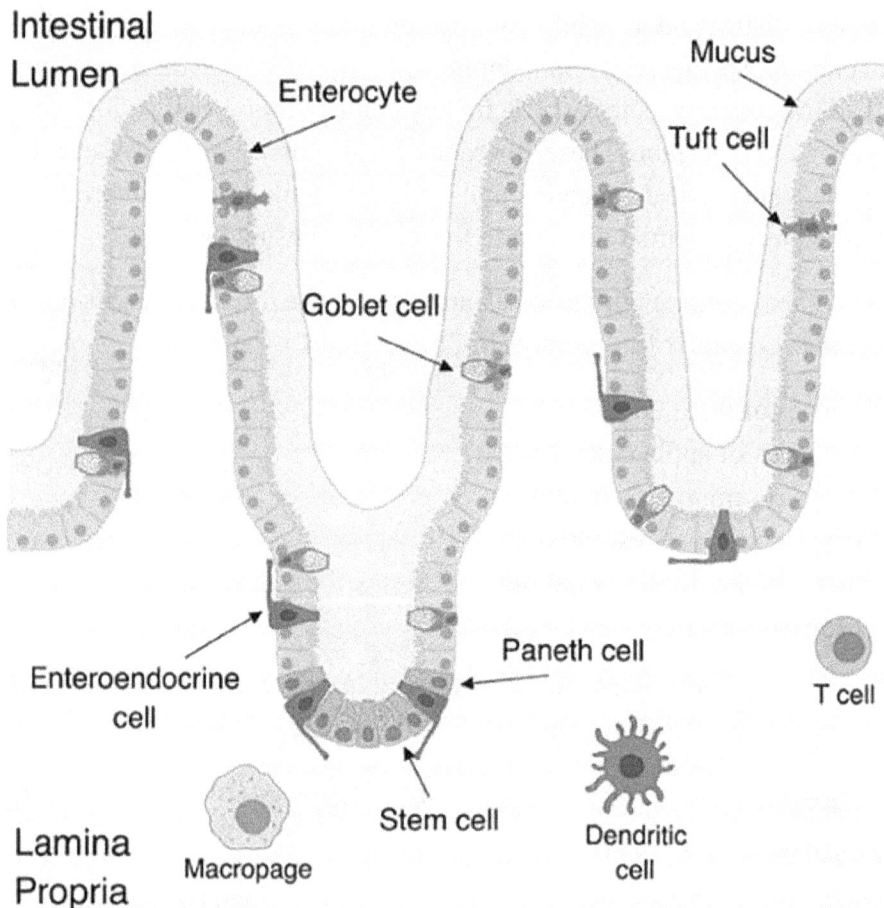

Probiotics and Synbiotics

Your mucosal immune system is primarily responsible for protecting the mucosal surfaces of the respiratory tract, nasal passages, GI tract, urinary tract, and even compartments of the eye. It acts as the first line of defense against harmful agents that enter the body and contact mucosal layers. Your GI tract is a highly microbiologically active ecosystem, and the bacteria present within it play a crucial role in mucosal immunity. Beneficial bacteria (probiotics) in the gut not only inhibit the growth of harmful bacteria but also stimulate the immune system through a complex network of molecular signals. Once ingested, probiotics interact with cells in the GI tract or immune cells and trigger the production of signaling molecules. This communication activates a variety of immune cells, including regulatory T cells that release IL-10—an anti-inflammatory cytokine.[160] They also increase mucins—gatekeepers of the mucosal barrier and tight junctions of the GI tract—and increase the number of Goblet cells to reinforce the mucus layer, which enhances intestinal barrier function.[161] In other words, activities are increased that improve the mucus layer in your intestines, kind of like putting over joints in drywall. Probiotics are critical for protection against pathogens and for supporting immune balance.

Synbiotics is a term used to describe a combination of prebiotics (substances, especially carbs, that act as food for probiotics) and probiotics. It is believed that synbiotics have a synergistic effect because the prebiotics help improve the survival and colonization of probiotics in the GI tract.[162] Synbiotics provide both probiotics and the "fuel" they need to function and thrive.

Beyond supplementing with a probiotic or synbiotic supplement, several factors influence the health and diversity of your gut microbiome. The following are foundational tips to help your probiotics thrive.

- *Consume fermented foods and beverages.* Consumed by humans for centuries, fermented foods and beverages employ an ancient food preservation technique whereby the food or beverage undergoes a controlled fermentation process. Bacteria or yeast break down carbs—sugars and starches—to ferment the food or beverage, thus altering its flavor and shelf life. Common fermented foods and beverages include yogurt, kefir, cider, sourdough bread, sauerkraut, kombucha, kimchi, and miso.

These foods are beneficial because they provide a variety of probiotics to encourage microbiome diversity.[163]

- *Eat plenty of fiber from vegetables, legumes, beans, and fruit.* Just like you, bacterial microbes require nutrition to stay viable. One source of nutrition for probiotics is fiber. Fiber can be digested by certain bacteria in the gut, which stimulates their growth and favorably alters the microbiome according to research.[164]

- *Reduce added sugar and unhealthy fats in your diet.* This one is common sense for general health, but sugar and unhealthy fats (PUFAs, trans, and saturated) also negatively impact your microbiome. Studies in animals show that high-fat or high-sugar diets contribute to dysbiosis and can increase brain inflammation and decrease brain function.[165] Additionally, surplus energy from dietary fat that is not needed for immediate energy production is stored in specialized cells called adipocytes. Excessive positive energy balance promotes the deposition of fats in cells other than adipocytes, leading to metabolic dysfunction and obesity.[166] Said another way, when you consume too much fat for your body to process, it runs out of normal storage space (adipocytes) and starts to store things anywhere else it can find space to do so. Since metabolism and weight are strongly correlated with aging and various health conditions, it is important to limit added sugar and unhealthy fats.

- *Manage stress.* Psychological stress affects virtually all aspects of human health. Your emotional and cognitive centers of the brain are linked to intestinal functions through the gut-brain axis. Simply put, the vagus nerve is like a telephone wire that connects the phone in the gut to the phone in the brain so the two organs can effectively communicate. The breakdown of food by gut bacteria produces metabolites (short-chain fatty acids) in the intestinal tract that are sensed by the vagus nerve—the longest and most complex of the twelve pairs of cranial nerves. In response to these intestinal metabolites, the vagus nerve delivers information to the brain. The vagus nerve is important for breathing, cardiovascular function, and inflammation control. Unfortunately, stress disrupts vagus nerve function, preventing it from performing these important tasks.[167]

- *Walk barefoot in the dirt.* Don't forget your skin microbiota. Walking barefoot allows direct contact with the soil, which has a positive effect on your mind and body. As you slowly stroll along the soil or grass with bare feet, you absorb some of the microbes in the ground. Even short-term direct contact with soil and plant materials can cause an immediate increase in beneficial microbes on your skin according to scientists.[168] One study even found that contact with microbes in the soil can make you feel happier.[169]

- *Reduce use of antimicrobial cleaners and only use antibiotics when absolutely necessary.* This is self-explanatory and was discussed earlier, but it is worth mentioning again. Antimicrobial cleaners kill both beneficial and potentially pathogenic organisms, and their overuse is suspected of contributing to antibiotic resistance. It isn't necessary to excessively wipe every surface you may touch with an antimicrobial cleaner. Exposure to microbes develops the immune system, so an overly sterile environment actually reduces immune system function. In addition, several studies have demonstrated that antibiotics can result in dysbiosis, and this disruption of the gut microbiome contributes to numerous diseases, including diabetes, obesity, inflammatory bowel disease, asthma, rheumatoid arthritis, depression, and autism.[170]

- *Take probiotics supplements.* To maintain a healthy and diverse microbiome, it is essential to take probiotic supplements. In fact, probiotics may be the single most important supplement a person can take. Look for a probiotic supplement with numbered strains listed on the bottle. These numbers are essential to ensure the correct probiotic strain is used for therapeutic benefits and clinical efficacy. For example, *Lactobacillus plantarum* 299v has been shown to effectively reduce IBS symptoms,[171] whereas administration of *L. plantarum* MF1298 can make IBS symptoms worse.[172] It is a good idea to rotate the probiotic you are taking to include different strains so that you maintain microbiome diversity. So, take one supplement for two to four weeks and then rotate to another probiotic that includes different strains for two to four weeks before returning to the original probiotic. Since you have cleansed and used natural antimicrobial agents, you'll want to take higher than maintenance doses of probiotics to repopulate and restore your gut microbiome.

Decades of research confirms that probiotics impact the immune system, and some are specifically beneficial for autoimmune and inflammatory disorders. Multiple randomized controlled trials show that improving gut-microbiome diversity and modifying harmful to beneficial microbe ratios in the gut help with gastrointestinal symptoms, inflammation, and autoimmune/autoinflammatory conditions like rheumatoid arthritis, ulcerative colitis, systemic lupus erythematosus, Sjogren's syndrome, systemic sclerosis, and multiple sclerosis.[173,174] With a systemic inflammatory condition involving compromised immune function, you need a systemic treatment. What better way to affect your whole body than to improve the core of your health, your gut, which educates the immune system and corrects compromised immune function. Maintaining an optimum balance of microbes in the gut can promote immune equilibrium where defenses against pathogens are safeguarded and tolerance to harmless antigens is preserved.

Several probiotic strains have been evaluated for their effects on people with autoimmune or autoinflammatory conditions. A few of them will be mentioned here so you can hopefully find a probiotic supplement that contains one or more of them.

Lactobacillus rhamnosus GG (LGG) regulates the immune system in several ways. One way is that it interferes with the inflammatory cascade to promote a healthy inflammatory response.[175]

Bifidobacterium bifidum BGN4 has been proven in various preclinical models to suppress allergic responses, diminish inflammation, and modulate immune cell activity; and to reduce IBS and eczema in humans.[176]

Bifidobacterium longum CECT 7347 may improve the digestion of gliadin, reducing its toxic and inflammatory effects in intestinal cells.[177,178,179] Taking *B. longum* CECT 7347 for three months, combined with a gluten-free diet, favorably altered the gut microbiome and improved immune responses in children.[180]

Bifidobacterium breve BR03 and *B. breve* B632 reduced the secretion of proinflammatory cytokines in children with celiac's disease.[181] The production of these cytokines increased three months after discontinuation of the probiotic, showing the need to continually take probiotics to maintain benefits.

Lactobacillus casei 01 (1 million CFU for eight weeks) decreased disease activity and improved the inflammatory response in people with rheumatoid arthritis.[182]

A synbiotic containing one billion probiotics (*L. casei, L. acidophilus, L. rhamnosus, L. bulgaricus, B. longum, B. breve, and S. thermophilus* with fructooligosaccharide and lactose-magnesium acetate-talc) significantly improved Th17 cells, and IL-17 and IL-23 gene expression in people with the autoinflammatory condition axial spondyloarthritis.

The commercial probiotic VSL#3, a blend of *Lactobacillus* and *Bifidobacteria*, improved the production of molecules important for immune equilibrium in a preclinical model of type 1 diabetes.[183] VSL#3 is considered a medical food and helps improve intestinal tight junctions to improve gut-barrier function, balances the gut microbiome, and helps regulate immune system signaling. It is considered helpful for allergies and other systemic diseases.[184]

Periodic fever, aphthous stomatitis, pharyngitis, and adenitis (PFAPA) syndrome is a childhood condition that causes repeated bouts of fever, mouth sores, sore throat, and swollen lymph nodes. A clinical trial found that ingestion of *Lactobacillus plantarum* HEAL9 and *Lactobacillus paracasei* 8700:2 significantly reduced the frequency of

PFAPA attacks.[185] Remarkably, 40 percent of the study participants had no attacks during the three-month trial.

A novel way to increase glutathione is to take the probiotic *Lactobacillus fermentum* ME-3. This unique probiotic supports healthy glutathione levels in four ways: 1) makes glutathione itself; 2) extracts available glutathione from its surrounding environments; 3) contains both glutathione peroxidase and glutathione reductase, providing it directly; and 4) recycles spent glutathione back into its active form (GSH).[186] This makes *Lactobacillus fermentum* ME-3 a complete glutathione system and powerhouse for fortifying your body's antioxidant defenses.

Typical dosage: Intensive repopulation after cleansing—at least 100 billion probiotics (CFUs) with eight or more strains, take daily with a meal for two to four weeks (VSL#3 is a great option); maintenance dose—at least ten billion probiotics (CFUs) with eight or more strains, daily with a meal; while using antimicrobials—at least ten billion probiotics (CFUs) with eight or more strains, two to four hours after antimicrobial use (may help reduce adverse effects of cleansing)
Cautions/Contraindications: None currently known
Potential adverse effects: Mild digestive discomfort

L-glutamine

Inside your gut are finger-like projectiles that control the passage of materials from your gut into the bloodstream called villi. The villi and microvilli capture and shuttle micronutrients towards tiny openings in your gut wall to allow them to be absorbed into the bloodstream. L-glutamine (glutamine) is an amino acid that plays a fundamental role in immune, digestive, muscular, and intestinal health. Beyond these important functions, glutamine helps maintain healthy gut-barrier function. It is a major nutrient for your gut cells, and depletion of this vital amino acid can lead to weakened villi function (leading to malabsorption), decreased expression of tight intestinal junctions, and increased intestinal permeability. Insufficient levels of glutamine significantly disrupts gut health.

The cells of the intestines are replaced every few days making it possible to heal the gut in a short period of time, perhaps only a few weeks. Glutamine enhances the production and survival of gut cells, speeding the time it takes to replace damaged cells—regrow and repair—that are allowing leakage of toxins and pathogens from the intestines to the bloodstream.[187] By supporting the health of your gut cells, glutamine helps promote tight intestinal junctions, reduce gut inflammation, and alleviate leaky gut.[188,189,190] Clinical research confirms that glutamine is important for digestive comfort and integrity. Ingestion of 5 g of glutamine, three times daily, for eight weeks, significantly improved leaky gut in people with IBS diarrhea caused by a GI infection.[191] Given its role in both gut integrity and immune function, glutamine is at the top of the list for supplements to heal the gut.

It is very difficult to consume enough glutamine in capsules, so it is most often taken in a free powder form that is mixed in a beverage. This may also be easier for your gut to digest and utilize.

Typical dosage: 5 g in a cold beverage, 1 to 4 times daily on an empty stomach
Cautions/Contraindications: Pregnancy, lactation, epilepsy and other convulsive disorders, liver cirrhosis, hepatic encephalopathy, anticonvulsant drugs
Potential adverse effects: Burping, bloating, constipation, cough, diarrhea, digestive discomfort, headache, musculoskeletal pain

Bovine Colostrum

The first form of breastmilk released by the mammals—including humans—after giving birth, colostrum is nutrient-dense and chock-full of antibodies, antioxidants, and growth factors. This super-nutrient is designed to promote growth and build and strengthen a newborn's immune system. When it comes to autoimmunity, colostrum contains immune factors (immunoglobulins IgA, IgG, IgM, proline-rich protein, lactoferrin) that regulate immune responses, growth factors (epidermal growth factor, transforming growth factor alpha and beta, insulin-like growth factor, vascular endothelial growth factor, and growth hormone) that repair damaged cells, and anti-inflammatory substances that fight inflammation.[192] Proline-rich protein regulates the thymus gland and inhibits the overproduction of immune cells, which is helpful for both autoimmunity and allergies. It can both stimulate a weakened immune system and stabilize it when it is hyperactive.[193,194] Lactoferrin helps maintain gut integrity and stability. Noting the benefits of colostrum for newborns, researchers have investigated bovine colostrum for such things as athletic performance, immune system function, and the maintenance of mucosal integrity.

Bovine colostrum (BC) is made from colostrum secreted by cows after giving birth. It has a long history of consumption by humans. Like human colostrum, it contains immune and growth factors, but in different amounts. Human colostrum has higher levels of most immune factors—BC is higher in IgG and contains IgG2, which is not present in human colostrum—and growth factors. Supplementation with BC has grown in popularity recently as additional research reveals its potential human health benefits.

One such benefit is to improve gut health and consequently immune health. Both animal and human studies prove that BC helps stimulate the growth of intestinal cells, strengthens the gut barrier, prevents leaky gut (even counteracting leaky gut caused by NSAIDs), and reduces inflammation in autoimmune diseases.[195,196,197,198] Autism spectrum disorder is partly linked to leaky gut and the subsequent production of autoantibodies. Taking BC with the probiotic *B. infantis* improved gut function and reduced the occurrence of aberrant behaviors associated with autism spectrum disorder in a clinical study.[199] More well-designed research is necessary in people with autoimmune and autoinflammatory conditions, but the emerging research is promising.

Like all supplements, quality is important for efficacy and safety. Inferior BC supplements will not do your body any good and leave you disappointed. Look for the following in a BC supplement: sourced from pasture-raised cows not treated with antibiotics or rBST, low-temperature pasteurization (flash pasteurized below 115 degrees F), collected within eight hours after calf birth, pure colostrum (no whey added), and high in IgGs (at least 20%). You should expect results in about three to four months.

Typical dosage: 2–5 g, one to four times daily, on an empty stomach; generally, start at 2 g, once a day and adjust as necessary
Cautions/Contraindications: Milk allergy, HIV
Potential adverse effects: Generally well tolerated orally, flatulence, nausea, vomiting

Quercetin

A plant flavonoid and potent antioxidant, quercetin is found in many common foods, such as apples, grapes, berries, onions, and tea. Quercetin stabilizes mast cells, preventing their release of chemicals including histamine, and also prevents intestinal cell toxicity.[200,201,202,203] Furthermore, quercetin enhances gut-barrier function because of its role in the assembly and expression of tight junction proteins and reverses gut dysbiosis.[204] This activity produces a sealing effect by connecting intestinal cells so nutrients can escape into the bloodstream, but larger molecules like toxins and pathogens can't escape the digestive tract. Experimental and animal research demonstrates that quercetin reverses leaky gut, heals the digestive tract, and restores depleted glutathione.[205,206,207,208] The takeaway is that you should eat fruits and vegetables rich in quercetin and consider taking a supplement (a better choice since getting therapeutic doses from food can be very difficult unless you like eating lots of onions) to fight leaky gut and dysbiosis.

Typical dosage: Quercetin—500 mg, two to three times daily; quercetin LipoMicel Matrix—250 mg, two to three times daily
Cautions/Contraindications: Pregnancy, lactation, bleeding disorders, kidney disorders, blood pressure lowering drugs, blood-thinning drugs, quinolone antibiotics, immunosuppressant drugs
Potential adverse effects: Headache, tingling of extremities

Larch Arabinogalactan (*Larix laricina, L. occidentalis*)

A starch-like fiber found in many plants, larch arabinogalactan (LA) is a complex carbohydrate (polysaccharide) that supports healthy immune system function. It is composed of galactose and arabinose in a 6:1 ratio, and a small amount of glucuronic acid. It is vigorously metabolized (fermented) by your gut microbiome, making it a prebiotic.[209] The major commercial source of LA is larch trees growing in North America. Human and preclinical studies confirm that LA enhances immune activity (increases NK cell and macrophage activity) and improves your body's ability to defend against viral infection.[210] The effect of LA was investigated in a simulator that models the human GI tract and microbiome. What the researchers concluded was that LA remarkably enhances gut-barrier function, decreases proinflammatory cytokine activity, and increases anti-inflammatory cytokine activity.[211] LA favorably modifies the gut microbiome, increasing *Bifidobacterium longum* better than other carbohydrate sources and improving the Firmicutes to Bacteroidetes ratio.[212,213] LA also increases the production of short-chain fatty acids, especially butyrate and propionate, which has further therapeutic benefits.[214] Lastly, LA interacts with microfold cells (M cells), which regulate immune function in the digestive tract.[215] Currently, the evidence suggests that LA can act as both an immune stimulator and immune suppressor, possibly based on your body's needs at the time.

Typical dosage: 1.5–2 g powder, on an empty stomach, two to three times daily

Cautions/Contraindications: Pregnancy, lactation, transplant recipients, immunosuppressive drugs

Potential adverse effects: Generally well tolerated orally, bloating, flatulence

Collagen (Marine or Bovine)

Collagen is the most abundant protein in the human body and there are twenty-eight types currently known in humans. It provides support, structure, and strength to your skin, connective tissue (ligaments and tendons), bones, teeth, and muscles. It is also present in your organs, blood vessels, and intestinal lining. Your body creates collagen daily from the amino acids obtained from protein-rich foods and supplements. Proline, glycine, and hydroxyproline are the main amino acids that comprise collagen and these amino acids group together to form protein fibrils in a triple helix structure. Vitamin C, zinc, copper, and manganese need to be present in your body in proper amounts to form this triple helix. Unfortunately, collagen production begins to decline in your mid-20s and by age 40 collagen is being depleted in your body faster than you can create it.[216] Since collagen is literally the "glue" that holds your body together, it is important to supplement with it beginning in your mid-to-late 20s.

Although twenty-eight types of collagen exist in the human body, there are five main types that are most abundant. These include:

- **Type I**. Making up 90 percent of your body's collagen, this densely packed collagen provides structure for your skin, tendons, ligaments, and bones. Type I collagen is the most abundant collagen in healthy intestines, followed by Type II and V.[217]
- **Type II**. This collagen is found in elastic cartilage and provides joint support.
- **Type III**. Found in muscles, arteries, and hollow organs (like your intestines), this collagen type aids wound healing, promotes skin elasticity, and helps regulate inflammatory processes.
- **Type IV**. Unlike Types I, II, and III, Type IV collagen doesn't form a fibrous triple helix structure. Instead, it creates a web-like pattern and makes up the thin outside layer of cells in the skin, liver, kidneys, and other internal organs.
- **Type V**. A unique type of collagen that helps form cell surfaces, this type of collagen is found in the cornea of your eyes, skin, and hair, and required for placental development during pregnancy.

Most people know that collagen supports their hair, skin, nails, joints, bones, and connective tissues, but few realize it's importance when it comes to gut health. Collagen aids gut health because it supplies large amounts of conditional amino acids—glycine, proline, and glutamine—that support gut microbiome balance and gut barrier integrity. Essential amino acids are those you must get from diet because your body doesn't create them. Nonessential amino acids can be made by the body, while conditional amino acids are those that become essential during periods of stress or illness. Collagen also reduces intestinal inflammation by supporting healthy gut-immune responses, largely due to its glutamine content.[218,219] Consequently, collagen is an important supplement to help heal and seal a damaged GI tract and allow your digestive system to get back to healthy functioning.

Of the over 300 different amino acids known, your body uses twenty—eleven nonessential and nine essential—to make the proteins required to sustain life. Seven conditionally essential amino acids—arginine, cysteine, glutamine, glycine, proline, serine, tyrosine—become essential when the body is overwhelmed by severe stress, illness, or injury, or simply can't keep up with nonessential amino acid production. Glutamine is fundamental to gut health because of its involvement in gut barrier integrity. The primary amino acid in collagen, glycine helps rebuild the lining of the GI tract. Proline is another amino acid abundant in collagen and it facilitates nutrient absorption and helps seal and heal the GI tract. In other words, collagen is packed with conditional amino acids that become essential when your gut needs repair.[220,221] Together, the amino acids in collagen mend damaged cells lining the GI tract and help restore intestinal integrity (reduce leaky gut). Since virtually everyone has some spectrum of leaky gut, collagen is a valuable supplement to take.

Furthermore, collagen strengthens the gut by providing more resistance to elastic stretch.[222] Resistance to stretch is important because if your gut stretches excessively too often it can gradually wear out the tight junctions and allow intestinal cells to become misaligned or spaced further apart, leading to leaky gut. A clinical study found that supplementing with 10 grams of collagen, twice daily, markedly reduced bloating and mild digestive symptoms without implementing any other lifestyle or dietary modifications among healthy women reporting regular digestive issues (bloating, flatulence, acid reflux, stomach pain, and irregular bowel movements).[223] The improvements were observed within six weeks of beginning supplementation, showing that collagen takes only a few short weeks to promote improved gut health. In addition, many people anecdotally report that taking a collagen supplement heals their leaky gut (occurring anywhere from three to twelve weeks after beginning supplementation).

While there are many collagen supplements to choose from, you need to choose a high-quality supplement to experience benefits. Some features to look for include: multiple collagen types (especially Types I and III; preferably at least five types of collagen); high tripeptide content (collagen is long chains of amino acids that need to be snipped up to be absorbable, which is what tripeptides are); no unnecessary fillers, artificial sweeteners, or flavors; grass-fed bovine or marine collagen from wild-caught fish; and, if possible, with other ingredients like vitamin C, biotin, and hyaluronic acid.

Typical dosage: Hydrolyzed collagen with average tripeptide content (15%–30%)—10–20 g, in two to three divided doses, daily; hydrolyzed collagen with 60%+ tripeptide content—3–6 g, in two to three divided doses, daily

Cautions/Contraindications: None currently known

Potential adverse effects: Generally well tolerated orally, rarely nausea, upset stomach, diarrhea, and flatulence

Deglycyrrhizinated Licorice Root, DGL (*Glycyrrhiza glabra*)

Primarily used to repair your gut lining by replenishing the GI mucus barrier, deglycyrrhizinated licorice root (DGL) is a special form of licorice root extract that has had the glycyrrhizin removed. This is because glycyrrhizin can raise blood pressure. DGL is used for a variety of ulcerative conditions of the GI tract from mouth to colon (canker sores, peptic ulcers, inflammatory bowel disease). Unlike antacids, DGL does not reduce stomach acidity. Instead, it stimulates the normal defense mechanisms that prevent ulceration and triggers the healing of already damaged mucus membranes. It does so by increasing blood supply to the damaged area, expanding the number of cells producing mucus, enhancing the amount of mucus produced by cells, and extending the lifespan of intestinal cells.[224,225] Licorice also increases the abundance of bacteria known to promote human health in the gut microbiome (*Bifidobacterium* spp., *Lactobacillus* spp., and Bacteroides spp.), while simultaneously diminishing harmful bacteria (*Citrobacter freundii* and *Klebsiella pneumoniae*).[226] Moreover, it increases butyrate- and propionate-producing bacterial species. Altogether, clinical experience and research verify that DGL improves gut-microbiome diversity and health, soothes the digestive tract, reduces inflammation, and improves intestinal cell function.

Typical dosage: One to two 380 mg chewable tablets before meals
Cautions/Contraindications: Pregnancy, lactation
Potential adverse effects: Generally well tolerated orally, nausea, vomiting

Marshmallow Root (*Althaea officinalis*)

Marshmallow root has a long history of medicinal use dating back to ancient Greek and Egyptian times. It is high in mucilage—a sap-like substance produced by plants—that helps coat the digestive tract. Interestingly, marshmallow candy got its name because confectioners used to use the mucilage from this plant's roots to make marshmallows. Mucilage acts similarly to the natural mucus barrier found in your GI tract, which works together with intestinal cells to maintain gut-barrier function. By coating the GI tract, marshmallow root helps reduce gut inflammation, improves gut-barrier integrity, promotes bowel regularity, and promotes healing of GI ulcers.

Typical dosage: 480 mg, twice daily, on an empty stomach
Cautions/Contraindications: Bleeding disorders, prior to surgery, lithium
Potential adverse effects: Generally well tolerated orally, stomachache

Slippery Elm Bark (*Ulmus rubra*)

Another restorative herb for the GI tract, slippery elm bark is one of the oldest herbal medicines used in North America. It works for GI problems in three ways: soothing the digestive tract, balancing the gut microbiome, and reducing inflammation. Like marshmallow root, slippery elm bark contains mucilage, which coats the tissues of the GI tract and allows them to heal. Having an ulcer-healing herb like this is important with leaky gut because the GI tract can become so inflamed that small ulcers can form. One clinical study found that slippery elm significantly improves GI irritation when combined with peppermint oil and DGL.[227] Acting as a prebiotic, slippery elm promotes a balanced and diverse gut microbiome.[228] The herb also reduces inflammation by decreasing proinflammatory cytokine production.[229] Slippery elm is another medicinal herb worth including because of its multilayered effects on gut health.

Typical dosage: Alcohol-free slippery elm tincture, as instructed on the product label, on an empty stomach
Cautions/Contraindications: Pregnancy, lactation
Potential adverse effects: Generally well tolerated orally

Aloe Juice, Extract, or Gel (*Aloe vera*)

Known for its soothing effects for sunburns, aloe vera has similar soothing effects on the GI tract when ingested. It has been used medicinally for thousands of years and is still popular today. Aloe vera is often consumed to aid overall digestion and improve nutrient absorption. Preclinical research shows that consuming aloe vera gel (not the kind intended topically for sunburns) enhanced the expression of tight junctions in the intestines to improve gut-barrier integrity.[230] Aloe vera, in its various edible forms, may support overall digestive health.

Typical dosage: As instructed on the product label on an empty stomach; studies have used 50 mL, four times daily, or 60 mL, twice daily
Cautions/Contraindications: Do not use aloe latex
Potential adverse effects: Generally well tolerated orally, stomachache, diarrhea

N-Acetyl Cysteine

As mentioned previously, ferroptosis is strongly correlated with gut health, which means it also impacts immune health. It plays an important role in regulating oxidative stress—an imbalance between free radicals (reactive oxygen species and reactive nitrogen species) and your body's ability to efficiently detoxify these free radicals with antioxidants—and inflammatory responses. Specifically, ferroptosis involves the inability to clear lipid peroxide (oxidation products created when fat cells are damaged by free radicals), the presence of redox-active iron (iron involved in electron transfers, which triggers oxidative stress through the formation of reactive oxygen species), and the oxidation of phospholipids containing polyunsaturated fatty acids (PUFAs).[231] This is one reason that a diet rich in PUFAs is inflammatory. PUFAs are oxidized more readily than saturated or monounsaturated fats, so greater levels of PUFAs increase ferroptosis. Contrarily, saturated and monounsaturated fats inhibit ferroptosis.[232] Abnormal cell death is a hallmark of ferroptosis. Abnormal cell death and the inadequate clearance of dead cells leads to exposure to intracellular contents that activate the immune system. In contrast to programmed cell death, where intracellular contents do not spill onto surrounding cells and cause harm, ferroptosis is an explosive death that leaves a clutter of cellular fragments in circulation, triggering an inflammatory response. The presence of this cellular debris and accumulation of cell waste materials may initiate and promote autoimmune disease. Some researchers suspect that ferroptosis is the leading cause of autoimmune reactions due to the abnormal cell death and subsequent exposure to contents inside dead cells that it causes.[233] Oxidative stress occurs in many autoimmune and autoinflammatory conditions.[234,235] Prolonged oxidative stress can lead to cell and tissue damage and increases the risk of chronic health conditions.

To combat oxidative stress, your body must activate endogenous cellular antioxidant systems, inhibit production of free radicals, or scavenge and neutralize free radicals with antioxidants. One of the key endogenous antioxidants to fight oxidative stress is glutathione. Glutathione is a powerful antioxidant found in every cell in your body, created from the amino acids glycine, glutamate, and cysteine. It serves many important functions, including making DNA, aiding immune function, helping create enzymes, regenerating antioxidant vitamins C and E, removing mercury from the brain, assisting normal cell death (apoptosis), supporting the liver and gallbladder in dealing with fats, forming sperm cells, stimulating or inhibiting immune responses to control inflammation, and, of course, neutralizing some free radicals. Glutathione levels can be reduced in your body by several factors, including nutrition, toxins, stress, and aging. Low levels are also observed in many autoimmune and chronic inflammatory conditions.[236]

Several readily available supplements appear to inhibit ferroptosis, such as N-acetyl cysteine (NAC), berberine, melatonin, red clover, and quercetin.[237,238,239,240,241,242] NAC is a precursor to the production of glutathione commonly used to help expel thick mucus from the lungs and to treat acetaminophen overdose. It also possesses antioxidant, anti-inflammatory, and immune-modulating properties. It has even been used clinically to improve cell-mediated immune function and counteract influenza.[243] NAC readily crosses the cell membrane where it is converted to cysteine and then glutathione. Because of this, it is a very efficient way to replenish glutathione stores inside cells.

Knowing the role of ferroptosis and oxidative stress in systemic lupus erythematosus (SLE) disease, researchers evaluated the effects of NAC supplementation in a randomized, double-blind, controlled trial.[244] Eighty people with SLE were divided into two groups: forty participants received 600 mg of NAC, three times daily, whereas forty participants in the control group received only standard therapies. After taking NAC for three months, the NAC group experienced significant improvement in SLE symptoms. The key finding of this study is that NAC supplementation successfully reduces SLE symptoms. However, additional findings can be extrapolated, including that NAC at least partly worked by reducing oxidative stress and inhibiting ferroptosis.

Amazingly, preclinical research suggests that NAC ingestion protects against disruption of intestinal tight junctions and barrier function as well.[245] This makes sense since oxidative stress damages intestinal cells, leading to holes in intestinal barriers. To summarize the NAC research, you could say that it protects cells against premature death by shoring up your antioxidant defenses. Subsequently, this protects other cells from "shrapnel" scattered into healthy cells during ferroptotic death. So, NAC is certainly worthy of trying for its effects on inflammation, immunity, oxidative stress, and ferroptosis.

Typical dosage: 600 mg, three times daily (maximum of 2,400 mg/day)

Cautions/Contraindications: NAC allergy, bleeding disorders, prior to surgery, blood pressure lowering drugs, blood-thinning drugs, activated charcoal, chloroquine

Potential adverse effects: Generally well tolerated orally up to 2,400 mg daily, diarrhea, heartburn, nausea, vomiting, loss of appetite, dry mouth

Berberine

An alkaloid compound found in many plants, such as European barberry, goldenseal, and Oregon grape, berberine boasts a host of human health benefits. Research shows that it is antibacterial, anti-inflammatory, balances blood sugar and insulin, promotes a healthy cholesterol profile, reduces high blood pressure, combats obesity, and favorably alters the gut microbiome.[246,247,248,249,250,251,252] Emerging research also suggests that it may be beneficial to manage rheumatoid arthritis because of its alteration of multiple immune signaling pathways involved in joint inflammation.[253,254]

When it comes to berberine and ferroptosis, berberine protects cell viability by inhibiting abnormal cell death and reducing the production of reactive oxygen species within cells.[255,256] Furthermore, it reduces the oxidation of fats (lipid peroxidation). Ferroptosis requires iron to react with PUFAs, generating excessive reactive oxygen species and oxidizing fats. Berberine interferes with this process and thus impedes ferroptosis. By doing so, berberine can preserve cells that make up vital tissues in the body and help maintain their ability to reproduce.

As a side benefit, berberine regulates the production of and mimics the action of a hormone called glucagon-like peptide 1 (GLP-1),[257,258] which means berberine helps manage glucose more efficiently and can result in weight loss. Blood sugar levels rise after eating, triggering the release of GLP-1, which enhances the secretion of insulin to move glucose from the blood and into your cells. It also suppresses glucagon secretion (glucagon is a hormone that increases blood sugar levels to prevent it from dropping too low, causing your liver to convert stored glucose into usable forms that are released into the bloodstream), delays emptying of food from the stomach, and increases satiety.[259] In addition to the metabolic effects berberine produces through GLP-1 alterations, restoration of GLP-1 secretion protects colon cells from damage, dysfunction, and destruction caused by mitochondrial stress responses.[260] This effect is important because mitochondrial stress contributes to dysbiosis and reduced production of short-chain fatty acids. Consequently, berberine helps protect gut health too! If that wasn't enough reason to take a berberine supplement, it also promotes healthy lipid profiles—reduces low-density lipoprotein (LDL) cholesterol, total cholesterol, triglycerides, and apolipoprotein B, while increasing high-density lipoprotein (HDL) cholesterol.[261] Interestingly, a systematic review found that berberine's effects on HDL cholesterol are more pronounced in women than in men, suggesting its effects may be sex specific.[262] Two more appealing findings are that berberine increases testosterone in men and helps relieve polycystic ovary syndrome (PCOS) in women.[263,264,265,266] The most effective dose for the above benefits seems to be 500 mg, three times daily. Berberine is a powerful natural molecule that has massive potential to aid the regulation of key mechanisms and pathways involved in human health.

Typical dosage: 400–600 mg, two to three times daily, with meals
Cautions/Contraindications: Pregnancy, lactation, cyclosporine, diabetes drugs, metformin, blood-thinning drugs, blood pressure lowering drugs, CNS depressant drugs, benzodiazepines, barbiturates, dextromethorphan, statins, immunosuppressive meds
Potential adverse effects: Generally well tolerated orally, abdominal pain or distension, diarrhea, constipation, flatulence, nausea, vomiting

Essential Oils

It is clear that essential oils are excellent antimicrobial agents, but emerging research suggests that they can also favorably change the gut microbiome and may possess prebiotic-like properties. A preclinical model found that emulsions containing summer savory, parsley, or rosemary essential oil acted as prebiotics to improve the gut microbiome, when taken with L-carnitine.[267] A mixture of bitter orange essential oil and grape hydrolat favored an increase in beneficial bacteria while simultaneously reducing pathogenic fungi, improving microbiome balance in animals.[268] Another study found that sweet orange essential oil—or isolated constituents found in the oil, including limonene, linalool, and citral—increased the abundance of *Lactobacillus* in the intestinal tract of mice.[269] Limonene was the most effective and also stimulated the production of short-chain fatty acids. Remarkably, both inhalation and feeding of sweet orange essential oil to mice increased the diversity of intestinal microflora (increased the abundance of Bacteroidetes and *Lactobacillus*).[270] Inhalation also improved immunoglobulins and immune activity. A significant increase in gut microflora diversity and short-chain fatty acids-producing bacteria (*Anaerostipes butyraticus, Butyrivibrio fibrisolvens, Clostridium jejuense, Eubacterium uniforme*, and *Lactobacillus lactis*) and simultaneous reduction in abundance of pathogens was observed when mice were administered patchouli essential oil.[271] A clinical trial evaluated ingestion of peppermint essential oil in children aged 7 to 12 with functional abdominal pain.[272] Ingesting the oil promoted improvements in the Firmicutes/Bacteroidetes ratio. The available evidence implies that essential oils have a positive effect on the gut microbiome despite their potent antimicrobial properties. Exactly how to use these oils for this purpose is not yet understood, so it may require some experimentation.

Typical dosage: Add 1 drop each of sweet orange, tangerine, peppermint, and patchouli essential oil to a "0" size capsule (only ingest pure, unadulterated essential oils), fill the rest with carrier oil (MCT, olive, black cumin seed, or avocado oil), and take morning and evening with a meal

Cautions/Contraindications: Iron-deficiency anemia, cyclosporine, caffeine

Potential adverse effects: Generally well tolerated orally, burp back (eructation), abdominal pain, nausea, vomiting, diarrhea

Genetics, Methylation, MTHFR, and Your Gut

Genetics is the study of heritable changes in gene activity or function due to the direct alteration of the DNA sequence. In contrast, epigenetics is the study of changes in gene activity or function that are not associated with any change of the DNA sequence itself. In other words, the way genes express—how your body reads your DNA—without changing the actual recipe contained in the DNA. Remarkably, all human beings share 99.9% of genetic information. The remaining 0.1% is what makes each of us unique and determines physical characteristics (phenotype) as well as how we respond to environmental factors. All human cells contain basically the same DNA (instructions for the creation and operation of cells), or genetic information. DNA consists of four nucleotide bases: cytosine (C), guanine (G), adenine (A), and thymine (T). DNA provides the instructions, but proteins carry out the functions. Areas within DNA sequences known as genes contain the information necessary for producing proteins. A controlled mechanism produces these proteins.

Whether a cell expresses as a liver, heart, bone, etc. cell depends on what sections of the gene are methylated—the transfer of a methyl group (one carbon and three hydrogen atoms) onto the C5 position of the cytosine to form 5-methylcytosine. Considering DNA methylation in comparison to baking may help in understanding this complex process. Even though you have the same basic ingredients—flour, sugar, baking soda, salt, a leavening agent, vegetable oil, and milk—whether these ingredients become bread, cake, or pancakes depends on the recipe you follow. Similarly, your body changes cell function based on what "recipe" is followed based on DNA methylation.

Methylation is a vital process not only for gene expression but to make healthy cells and neurotransmitters, remove toxins, fight infections, and combat oxidative stress. If a DNA section is hypermethylated no further methylation can occur, but if a section in hypomethylated, methylation can occur. When a section of DNA is methylated, your body function changes, potentially affecting your health in many ways. Demethylation involves the removal of a methyl group and also alters cellular function. Cellular structure and function are determined by what cells are turned on or off by methylation inside any given cell. One way to view methylation is to consider the body in terms of its complexity with various gears and switches that need to be functioning properly for optimum health to occur. Methylation and demethylation are the ways that your body controls the turning of gears and what biological switches are turned up or down, on or off. Typically, methylation turns genes "off" and demethylation turns genes "on."

Your methylation cycle relies upon the enzyme methylenetetrahydrofolate reductase (MTHFR). The MTHFR gene instructs the body to make this enzyme, which is required to convert folate (vitamin B9) into an active and usable form (5-methyltetrahydrofolate; 5-MTHF). This enzyme also breaks down the amino acid homocysteine. Additionally, methylation is the processes used to convert B vitamins (folate and B12) into S-adenosyl methionine (SAM), which is further used to balance neurotransmitters (like serotonin and dopamine) levels. SAM is also important for DNA protection, energy production, and the break down of histamine. Mutations in this gene can slow down the methylation cycle and may contribute to a variety of health conditions—autism spectrum disorder, depression, ADHD, migraines, glaucoma, certain types of cancer, cardiovascular disease, miscarriage, and more.[273,274,275,276,277]

You have two MTHFR genes, inheriting one from each of your parents. Mutations can involve one gene (heterozygous) or both (homozygous) depending on what you inherit from each parent. Common variants of MTHFR mutations include C677T, C665C, A1298C, and A1286C. More than twenty-five percent of Hispanics and about ten to fifteen percent of North American Caucasians are estimated to be homozygous for the MTHFR 677 TT variant, while it is less common in people of African descent.[278,279] However, some experts believe MTHFR mutations are significantly underreported and underdiagnosed because they are not routinely screened for and believe that it is more likely that forty to sixty percent of the population carries an MTHFR mutation.

People who are TT homozygous usually have higher homocysteine levels and lower blood levels of folate. The A1298C and A1286C mutations—both heterozygous and homozygous—are not linked to increased homocysteine levels unless they are combined with a C677T mutation.

As additional links between MTHFR mutations and health conditions are discovered, more and more individuals are learning that they carry a mutation. People with an MTHFR mutation or methylation issues are more likely to experience leaky gut and suffer from severe leaky gut symptoms. This is because anything that causes stress to your body can disrupt methylation, particularly if you already have impaired methylation due to an MTHFR mutation. When you are stressed, your methylation cycle must work harder to perform its functions, which requires more B vitamins to get the work done. That's why we are often told to replenish B vitamins when recovering from stress. What resides in your gut microbiome and whether intestinal integrity is maintained has a significant impact on your methylation cycle and downstream the expression of your genes and body functions. On the other hand, methylation produces the SAM necessary to make new healthy cells that line the GI tract and maintain intestinal integrity. Consequently, healing your gut is vital to improving methylation, and conversely supporting methylation is important for gut and overall health.

The steps outlined in this book will help to attack bacteria and their production of endotoxins, help you deal with existing endotoxins, and promote a gut environment that optimizes DNA methylation. Below are additional supplements to support healthy methylation when an MTHFR mutation is present.

As stated earlier, 5-MTHF is the active form of folate and the form that people with MTHFR mutations should take. Your body is incapable of directly using folate, necessitating the conversion of folate to methylfolate so it can be used. It is responsible for methylation throughout your body. People with MTHFR mutations do not convert folic acid—a synthetic form of folate found in fortified foods and many multivitamins—to methylfolate, making folate insufficiency or deficiency common.

Typical dosage: L-methylfolate as (6S)-5-methyltetrahydrofolate—may be labeled as (6S)-5-methyltetrahydrofolic acid, calcium salt; L-methylfolate; (6S)-5-methyltetrahydrofolic acid, monosodium salt; L-methyltetrahydrofolate, glucosamine salt, 1–15 mg daily in the morning, with B12; take according to symptoms—fatigue/lethargy (1–4 mg), neuropathy, pins and needles (3 mg), psychological issues (7.5–15 mg; 15 mg appears to be more effective), cognitive symptoms, poor memory, brain fog (5–6 mg), GI symptoms (7.5–15 mg)

Cautions/Contraindications: Seizure disorders, B12 deficiency, cancer drugs, barbiturates, antiseizure drugs, pyrimethamine

Potential adverse effects: Generally well tolerated orally, abdominal cramps, nausea, diarrhea, bitter taste, insomnia or sleep disturbance, anxiety, anger, irritability, hyperactivity, headache or migraine, confusion, rash, acne, achy joints or muscles

Vitamin B12 is an essential vitamin important for red blood cell formation, cell metabolism, nerve function, and DNA protection. It augments the function of other B vitamins as well. Cyanocobalamin—the synthetic form found in fortified foods and many multivitamins—needs to be converted to its active form (methylcobalamin) for your body to use it. B12 levels may be high in people with MTHFR mutations because inadequate folate means that B12 doesn't have enough folate to work with. Three natural forms of B12 are available: methylcobalamin, hydroxocobalamin, and adenosylcobalamin, all of which are bioidentical to B12 forms naturally occurring in humans and animal foods. Genetic mutations (polymorphisms) in B12-related pathways may affect the bioavailability, cellular uptake, and tolerance to the various forms.

Typical dosage: Methylcobalamin, hydroxocobalamin, or adenosylcobalamin (preferably sublingual tablets) based on gene status—see table below, 1–5 mg (1,000–5,000 mcg); You can also find supplements with all three forms—which may produce faster clinical results and help offset polymorphisms in B12-related pathways—that are paired with L-methylfolate

Cautions/Contraindications: None currently known

Potential adverse effects: Well tolerated orally

COMT V158M Point Mutation	Vitamin D Receptor Taq	Tolerated B12 Form(S)
- -	+ + (TT)	methyl, hydroxo, adenosyl
- -	+ - (Tt)	methyl, hydroxo, adenosyl (lower doses)
- -	- - (tt)	hydroxo, adenosyl
+ -	+ +	methyl, hydroxy, adenosyl (lower doses)
+ -	+ -	hydroxo, adenosyl

+ -	- -	hydroxo, adenosyl
+ +	+ +	hydroxo, adenosyl
+ +	+ -	hydroxo, adenosyl
+ +	- -	hydroxo

Catechol-O-Methyltransferase (COMT) is one of several enzymes that degrade dopamine, epinephrine, and norepinephrine. Additionally, it transfers methyl groups—introduces a methyl group to the catecholamine (dopamine, epinephrine, and norepinephrine), which is donated by SAM. A point mutation in the COMT gene called V158M (or rs4680) is well-researched and associated with differences in intelligence, personality, sensitivity to pain, and disease risk.

The vitamin D receptor (VDR) gene provides instructions for making a protein called VDR, which is the cellular target for vitamin D. The VDR binds to the active form of vitamin D (calcitriol), triggering a cascade of biological activity. Single nucleotide polymorphism (SNP) located in the VDR gene Taq I (rs731236) can alter responses to vitamin D and is linked to various adverse health conditions.

A compound consisting of glycine with three attached methyl groups, trimethylglycine (betaine anhydrous) acts as a potent methyl donor. Beyond being involved in DNA methylation, it also converts homocysteine into methionine—an essential amino acid and a precursor to SAM production involved in the DNA methylation cycle. Trimethylglycine is especially valuable for those with mutations that lead to high homocysteine levels.

Typical dosage: Children 2–5 years—500 mg, two to three times daily; children 6–12 years—1,000–2,000 mg, twice daily; teens/adults—1,000–3,000 mg, two to three times daily
Cautions/Contraindications: High cholesterol
Potential adverse effects: Generally well tolerated orally, diarrhea, GI discomfort, nausea, vomiting, body odor, elevated cholesterol levels

Furthermore, those with an MTHFR mutation should take NAC (to support glutathione production and detoxification) and take magnesium (acts as a cofactor in the methylation cycle) and glutathione (people with MTHFR mutations are more likely to be deficient in this key antioxidant and therefore experience health related problems associated with its depletion).

There are many forms of magnesium to choose from, each of which can have a different effect and outcome when taken as a dietary supplement. Each should be taken as directed on the supplement or product label.

Form	Benefits/Usage
Bicarbonate	pH balance
Bisglycinate	Intestinal health, muscle relaxation, deficiency, sleep, heart health, blood sugar, mental health, mood
Chloride	Digestion
Citrate	Constipation, deficiency, migraine
Glycinate	Relaxation, calming, sleep, inflammation, mental health
Malate	Energy, deficiency, muscle soreness
Orotate	Heart health, physical performance
Oxide	Digestion, migraine
Sucrisominal	Deficiency
Sulfate	Muscle aches, stress
Taurate	Blood pressure, blood sugar
Threonate	Cognition, nervous system support, mood

Typical dosage: See above table (bisglycinate, citrate, Sucrisominal, or malate may be the best options)

Cautions/Contraindications: Heart block, kidney disease, levodopa/carbidopa, aminoglycoside, tetracycline, and quinolone antibiotics, bisphosphonates, digoxin, ketamine, potassium-sparing diuretics, sevelamer, muscle relaxants, sulfonylureas

Potential adverse effects: Generally well tolerated orally, diarrhea, stomach upset, nausea, vomiting

While you wouldn't normally take all these supplements to support a healthy gut at the same time—at least at the therapeutic dosage—you are likely to see the most success if you take a supplement from each area: replenish (probiotics, essential oils), strengthen (glutamine, quercetin, colostrum, LA, collagen), restore (DGL, marshmallow root, slippery elm, aloe vera), protect against ferroptosis (NAC, berberine), and aid DNA methylation if necessary (methylfolate, active B12, trimethylglycine, NAC, magnesium, glutathione). The human gut is highly complex, but it is clear that total health follows gut health. Maintaining, or restoring, healthy gut function contributes to balanced immune function, improved mood, cognitive health, cardiovascular health, restorative sleep, efficient digestion, a healthy inflammatory response, and may prevent a host of chronic autoimmune, autoinflammatory, and other health conditions.

While the above focuses on balancing immune function when it is overactive, those who experience immunodeficiency require a different approach. Conventional treatment calls for drugs like antibiotics, immunoglobulin therapy, antivirals, or interferon. However, as with all pharmaceutical approaches, such treatments do not address the root cause of the issue and inevitably cause undesirable side effects.

A better approach to immunodeficiency is to strengthen the immune system at the cellular level by providing optimum levels of key micronutrients (vitamins and minerals), trace elements, cellular cofactors, and amino acids. Absorption of these nutrients requires a healthy gut. Below is a general guideline for providing these vital nutrients (amounts are daily), which should be adjusted according to your individual needs and preferably determined through blood work by a knowledgeable healthcare professional.

VITAMINS	
Vitamin C (Buffered forms with bioflavonoids)	1,000–5,000 mg
Vitamin D (Cholecalciferol D3)	2,000–5,000 IU
Vitamin K (K2, MK7)	50–150 mcg
Vitamin E (Mixed tocopherols)	200–600 IU
Beta-carotene (Mixed carotenoids)	2,000–8,000 IU
Vitamin B1 (Allithiamine)	25–100 mg
Vitamin B2 (Riboflavin-5-phosphate)	25–100 mg
Vitamin B3 (Nicotinamide Riboside)	25–100 mg
Vitamin B5 (Pantethine)	25–100 mg

Vitamin B6 (Pyridoxal-5-phosphate)	25–100 mg
Vitamin B7 (Biotin)	300–800 mcg
Vitamin B9 (L-Methylfolate)	400–1,000 mcg
Vitamin B12 (Methylcobalamin)	100–400 mcg
MINERALS	
Calcium (Citrate)	30–150 mg
Magnesium (Citrate, Bisglycinate)	200–500 mg
Potassium (Gluconate)	20–75 mg
TRACE ELEMENTS	
Zinc (Amino acid chelate, with quercetin)	15–45 mg
Manganese (Gluconate, Picolinate)	5–7 mg
Selenium (Selenomethionine)	100–200 mcg
Chromium (Picolinate)	50–200 mcg
Molybdenum (Amino acid chelate)	50–200 mcg
AMINO ACIDS & CELLULAR COFACTORS	
L-Arginine	0.5–1.5 g
L-Carnitine	0.5–1.5 g
L-Cysteine	0.5–1.5 g
L-Lysine	0.5–1.5 g
L-Proline	0.5–1.5 g
Inositol (Myo and D-Chiro; 40:1 ratio)	0.5–2 g
Coenzyme Q-10 (Ubiquinol)	50–300 mg
Quercetin	500 mg
Bioflavonoids	100–500 mg

When it comes to immune system cancers, one should work with an integrative physician or qualified healthcare professional to determine the best course of action. Although many natural options exist, much of the research for cancer and natural solutions is in its infancy. Moreover, multiple lifestyle adjustments will be necessary as cancer requires a targeted but broad and multifaceted approach.

5

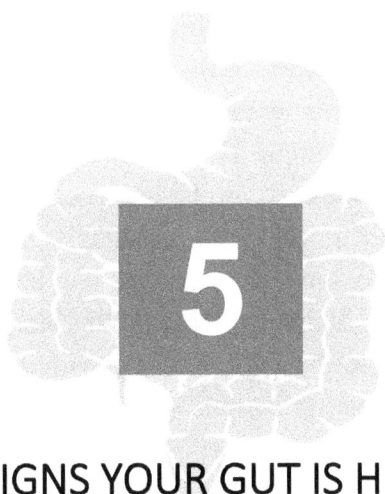

SIGNS YOUR GUT IS HEALING

Now that you've been empowered with a plethora of information about gut health and function and how you can support this, the obvious question is *how do I know if my gut is healing?* The gut-healing process can be a bumpy one. You may initially feel worse as toxins are mobilized, pathogens are eliminated (releasing toxic byproducts), and your gut adjusts to its new environment. You'll have ups and downs in the healing process. Stay committed! Don't let these bumps in the road derail your entire journey of healing your gut to heal your immune system.

Diagnostics Tests and Labs as a Sign of Gut and Immune Healing

Of course, there are diagnostics tests to evaluate the presence or absence of GI issues. One way to examine gut health is through a fecal (stool) test. In other words, your poop is examined for waste products or the balance of microbes present in your GI tract. A calprotectin test looks for the protein calprotectin in your stool, which can indicate inflammatory activity due to activated white blood cells. Specifically, it is used as a diagnostics tool for inflammatory bowel disease. Another stool test is the fecal occult blood test (fecal immunochemical test), which is a procedure used to determine whether there is bleeding in the GI tract. Blood in the GI tract can indicate bowel cancer or polyps in the rectum or colon. Screening for changes in your cell's genetic material (DNA), a stool DNA test is another colon cancer detection test. After your healthcare provider prescribes a stool DNA test, a sample collection kit is mailed to you. You collect a stool sample using the kit in the privacy of your own home and send it back in the prepaid, pre-addressed box. The stool sample is then analyzed in a laboratory. Certain DNA changes (mutations) are linked to cancer—both existing and probable. Cancerous cells and polyps (a small clumps of cells that form in the lining of the colon that could one day become cancerous) continuously shed cells with altered DNA into the stool. Very sensitive lab tests detect these DNA changes in people with an average risk of colon cancer and who have no current symptoms of colon cancer. If altered DNA is detected during the test, a colonoscopy is performed to confirm the test results. Lastly, a microbiome test examines the amount and types of microbes present in your gut.

Tests for zonulin and antibodies (occludin, actomysin, and lipopolysaccharides) are important because these two proteins regulate gut permeability. Abnormally high zonulin levels suggests that gut barrier is not performing well. The presence of the mentioned antibodies is a good indicator that your intestinal tight junctions are damaged, your gut lining is being destroyed, and you have leaky gut. Zonulin is tested with an enzyme-linked immunosorbent assay (ELISA) test. Antibodies are measured via a blood draw.

Breath tests are also used as GI diagnostics tools. One of the most common tests is the *H. pylori* breath test. If your health-care professional suspects you have an *H. pylori* infection, she may send you for this test. During the test, you swallow a capsule containing C-13 urea. If sufficient *H. pylori*—a bacterium associated with stomach ulcers and cancer—is present in the stomach the bacteria will react with the C-13 urea and produce gases that are detectable in your breath. Hydrogen and methane breath tests are used to detect lactose intolerance and small intestinal bacterial overgrowth (SIBO). Higher than normal amounts of hydrogen during the test may suggest undigested sugars, or lactose intolerance. The presence of both high methane and hydrogen are signs that the bacteria has entered the small intestine and is an indicator of SIBO.

Manometry is a diagnostic technique that shows whether your esophagus is working properly. During an esophageal manometry procedure, a small tube is inserted through the nose down through the esophagus. The tube detects vibrations from rhythmic muscle contractions, which are then graphed on a machine. Muscle contraction strength and coordination is determined during this procedure to rule out conditions that mimic GERD. Anorectal manometry involves the insertion of a catheter with a deflated balloon through the anus and into the rectum. The balloon is slowly inflated causing the rectum to contract and these contractions are measured by a machine. Anorectal manometry is primarily used to see if the anal sphincter muscles are working properly.

A barium test combines X-rays with a substance called barium that coats the GI tract and makes it more visible to a radiologist. There are multiple types of barium tests. The barium swallow test looks for abnormalities in the esophagus and upper stomach like ulcers, blockages, or growths. A second test, called the barium meal test, evaluates the esophagus, stomach, and beginning of the small intestine. Lastly, a barium enema can be used to observe the colon.

Endoscopic procedures, where a flexible tube or capsule-based camera is inserted into the GI tract, allow your physician to view the insides of the GI tract. There are many types of endoscopies, including the following:

- Gastroscopy, upper endoscopy: views of the esophagus, stomach, and upper small intestine (duodenum) through the mouth; commonly used to diagnose GERD, celiac disease, throat or stomach cancer, stomach ulcers, and Barrett's esophagus
- Sigmoidoscopy: views the lower colon through the anus; commonly used to diagnose causes of diarrhea, stomach pain, constipation, polyps, or bleeding

- Colonoscopy: views the entire large intestine through the anus; commonly used to diagnose large intestine abnormalities, inflammatory bowel disease, colorectal cancer, and polyps
- Proctoscopy: views the rectum and anal cavity through the anus; commonly used to screen for colorectal cancer
- Endoscopic retrograde cholangiopancreatography views the liver, pancreas, gallbladder, and bile duct through the mouth; commonly used to diagnose blockages, infection, or stones in the bile ducts, fluid leaks, tumors, or narrowing of the pancreas
- Capsule endoscopy: views the esophagus, stomach, small intestine, large intestine, and rectum via swallowing a camera capsule; commonly used to diagnose polyps, inflammatory bowel disease, ulcers, and tumors of the small intestine

Technology also allows viewing of the GI system virtually through a virtual colonoscopy. During this procedure, a CT scan produces cross-sectional images of the abdominal organs looking for abnormalities or changes. To improve image quality, a small tube (catheter) is inserted into the rectum to fill your colon with air or carbon dioxide. Some people choose this over traditional colonoscopy because it only takes about ten to thirty minutes and doesn't require sedation or insertion of a scope into the colon—but this does preclude tissue biopsies and the removal of polyps, which if found will require a colonoscopy anyway.

Another noninvasive test is an MRI scan. This test leverages powerful magnets and radio waves to create detailed three-dimensional images of your digestive organs. It is an effective way to detect appendicitis, inflammatory bowel disease, acute pancreatitis, and an obstructed bile duct (choledocholithiasis).

Blood tests could be used as an indicator of immune system healing, especially inflammatory markers. A comprehensive metabolic panel (basal metabolic panel) measures your metabolism, detecting levels of electrolytes and minerals in your blood. This provides a picture of how well your various organs are functioning. A complete blood count (CBC) can detect abnormalities in red or white blood cells, or clotting problems. Other routine tests measure inflammation, such as fibrinogen, haptoglobin, and albumin, but are not necessarily signs of an autoimmune condition. C-reactive protein (CRP) is a protein made by the liver and its level increases as inflammation increase in the body. Two tests can measure CRP in the blood: CRP and hs-CRP. hs-CRP is more sensitive than CRP, allowing for the ability to measure smaller increases in CRP levels. CRP level is frequently used as a marker for chronic inflammatory conditions, like lupus or rheumatoid arthritis, to assess heart disease or heart attack risk, and to check for infection. Erythrocyte sedimentation rate (ESR, sed rate) is a blood test used alongside other tests to monitor the progression of an inflammatory condition. Red blood cells (erythrocytes) gradually settle to the bottom of a tube when placed upright. Inflammation causes erythrocytes to clump together making them settle to the bottom more quickly. The farther the erythrocytes fall in the test tube, the greater the inflammatory response by your immune system. Some other inflammatory tests worth mentioning are the antinuclear antibodies (ANA) test, anti-cyclic citrullinated peptide (anti-CCP) antibodies test, and rheumatic factor (RF) test. Antinuclear antibodies attack your own healthy cells, specifically targeting the nucleus of cells. Finding ANA in your blood can indicate you have an autoimmune disorder, but keep in mind that many healthy people also have low levels of ANAs without any active autoimmune disorder.[280,281] An anti-CCP test looks for autoantibodies in the blood that are associated with rheumatoid arthritis. It is frequently performed in conjunction with an RF test. A RF test measures the amount of RF—proteins produced by your immune system that can attack healthy tissues—in your blood. High RF levels are associated with autoimmune conditions, but again, some people without an autoimmune condition also have abnormally high levels of RF. Neither an ANA nor RF test should be used as the sole determinant of an autoimmune disorder.

Symptomatic Signs of Gut Healing

Lab and test improvements are a good sign that your efforts to heal your gut and immune system are paying off. However, you don't need to perform diagnostics tests to know your gut is healing. You can also identify gut healing based on symptom improvements. Digestive issues—flatulence, bloating, heartburn, and constipation—are common, but not always present, with autoimmune and autoinflammatory conditions. This is particularly true if the trigger for your condition was an infection. Correction, or at a minimum diminishment, of digestive issues is a good sign that your gut health is improving.

Gut issues, especially leaky gut, are associated with food sensitivities. Partially digested food particles escape your gut and enter the bloodstream where they cause immune and inflammatory reactions. More systemic reactions like fatigue, headache, mood disturbance, and brain fog can also occur. Histamine intolerance is often cleared up as your gut and digestive processes improve. Finding that you can consume previously triggering foods without digestive or systemic issues is a signal your gut is healing.

Your quality of life can also improve. Chronic inflammation and immune attacks on self can lead to constant achiness, fatigue, lack of mental clarity, weight gain, and low overall energy and vitality. If you feel like your best, healthy self again with plenty of energy, a healthy mood, minimal soreness, and strong cognitive abilities, your gut is on the mend.

Eczema, psoriasis, rosacea, acne, rashes, and dandruff are all outward manifestations of an internal issue, poor gut health. Your microbiome and gut barrier play important roles in skin health. Your gut is in direct communication with your skin through the gut-skin access. This bidirectional communication aims to maintain skin homeostasis. As your gut heals, you'll likely see your skin problems clear up as well.

Pathogenic microbes in your gut try to hijack gut communication with the brain to manipulate you into eating foods that help them thrive. Microbes trick your gut into sending powerful signals to consume foods that they want and need. Yeast, like *Candida*, thrives on sugar; whereas *Bifidobacteria* prefer dietary fiber, and Bacteroidetes love fats. Too much yeast in the gut can lead to intense sugar cravings—making it more important to exterminate yeasts as part of your cleanse—that feeds the yeast and perpetuates a suboptimal gut.

Lastly, when your gut is healthy, your immune system is healthy. Maintaining a healthy gut and robust gut microbiome stabilizes immune responses, so pathogens are efficiently dealt with, and healthy cells and tissues left alone. A healthy gut teaches your immune system to better discriminate between pathogen and self, leading to reduced inflammation.

Keep in mind that gut and immune healing is not a constant forward march. You will have days with improvements and days of setbacks. The most important thing is to stay persistent in your efforts and not let setbacks become permanent by giving up. If you are consistent with lifestyle adjustments and use the right high-quality dietary supplements, you will see results. The longer you have had your condition and an unhealthy gut, the more difficult it will be and the longer it will take for you to see results. Your gut didn't become unhealthy overnight. It likely took years of exposure and lifestyle factors to develop. You can't expect overnight results. Commit to your health. It will be worth it! As your health is rejuvenated, you'll be restored to your best healthy self again. Regardless of your age, gender, or race, you can enjoy a longer, healthier, and higher quality of life.

REFERENCES

[1] Fasano A, Shea-Donohue T. Mechanisms of disease: the role of intestinal barrier function in the pathogenesis of gastrointestinal autoimmune diseases. *Nat Clin Pract Gastroenterol Hepatol.* 2005;2:416–422.

[2] Groschwitz KR, Hogan SP. Intestinal barrier function: molecular regulation and disease pathogenesis. *J Allergy Clin Immunol.* 2009;124:3–20.

[3] Tsurugizawa T, Uematsu A, Nakamura E, et al. Mechanisms of neural response to gastrointestinal nutritive stimuli: the gut-brain axis. *Gastroenterology.* 2009;137:262–273.

[4] Silva YP, Bernardi A, Frozza RL. The Role of Short-Chain Fatty Acids From Gut Microbiota in Gut-Brain Communication. *Front Endocrinol.* 2020 Jan 31;11:25.

[5] Dalile B, Van Oudenhove L, Vervliet B, et al. The role of short-chain fatty acids in microbiota-gut-brain communication. *Nat Rev Gastroenterol Hepatol.* 2019;16:461–478.

[6] Guo C, Hup YJ, Li Y, et al. Gut-brain axis: Focus on gut metabolites short-chain fatty acids. *World J Clin Cases.* 2022 Feb 26;10(6):1754–1763.

[7] Sender R, Fuchs S, Milo R. Revised estimates for the number of human and bacteria cells in the body. *PLoS Biol.* 2016 Aug;14(8):e1002533.

[8] Park SY, Hwang BO, Lim M, et al. Oral–Gut Microbiome Axis in Gastrointestinal Disease and Cancer. *Cancers (Basel).* 2021 May;13(9):2124.

[9] Zhu W, Wu Y, Liu H, et al. Gut–Lung Axis: Microbial Crosstalk in Pediatric Respiratory Tract Infections. *Front Immunol.* 2021;12:741233.

[10] Zhang D, Li S, Wang N, et al. The Cross-Talk Between Gut Microbiota and Lungs in Common Lung Diseases. *Front Microbiol.* 2020; 11: 301.

[11] van Meel ER, Jaddoe VWV, Bonnelykke K, et al. The role of respiratory tract infections and the microbiome in the development of asthma: A narrative review. *Pediatr Pulmonol.* 2017 Oct; 52(10): 1363–1370.

[12] Sinha S, Lin G, Ferenczi K. The skin microbiome and the gut-skin axis. *Clin Dermatol.* 2021 Sep-Oct;39(5):829-839.

[13] Bullman S, Pedamallu CS, Sicinska E, et al. Analysis of Fusobacterium Persistence and Antibiotic Response in Colorectal Cancer. *Science.* 2017;3586369:1443–8.

[14] Gao L, Xu T, Huang G, et al. Oral microbiomes: More and more importance in oral cavity and whole body. *Protein Cell.* 2018;9:488–500.

[15] Wade W.G. The oral microbiome in health and disease. *Pharmacol Res.* 2013;69:137–143.

[16] Joshipura KJ, Munoz-Torres FJ, Morou-Bermudez E, et al. Over-the-counter mouthwash use and risk of pre-diabetes/diabetes. *Nitric Oxide.* 2017 Dec 1;71:14-20.

[17] Preshaw PW. Mouthwash use and risk of diabetes. *Br Dent J.* 2018 Nov 23;225(10):923-926.

[18] Aagaard K, Ma J, Antony KM, et al. The placenta harbors a unique microbiome. *Sci Transl Med.* 2014 May 21;6(237):237ra65.

[19] Hill CJ, Lynch DB, Murphy K, et al. Evolution of gut microbiota composition from birth to 24 weeks in the INFANTMET Cohort. *Microbiome.* 2017 Jan 17;5(1):4.

20 Hoang DM, Levy EI, Vandenplas Y. The impact of Caesarean section on the infant gut microbiome. *Acta Paediatr.* 2021 Jan;110(1):60-67.

21 Walker WA. The importance of appropriate initial bacterial colonization of the intestine in newborn, child and adult health. *Pediatr Res.* 2017 Sep; 82(3): 387–395.

22 Jost T, Lacroix C, Braegger CP, et al. New insights in gut microbiota establishment in healthy breast fed neonates. *PLoS ONE.* 2012;7:e44595.

23 Koenig JE, Spor Am Scalfone N, et al. Succession of microbial consortia in the developing infant gut microbiome. *Proc Natl Acad Sci U S A.* 2011 Mar 15;108 Suppl 1(Suppl 1):4578-85.

24 Vijay A, Valdes Am. Role of the gut microbiome in chronic diseases: a narrative review. *Eur J Clin Nutr.* 2022;76:489-501.

25 Rothschild D, Weissbrod O, Barkan E, et al. Environment dominates over host genetics in shaping human gut microbiota. *Nature.* 2018;555:210-215.

26 Rowland I, Gibson G, Heinken A, et al. Gut microbiota functions: metabolism of nutrients and other food components. *Eur J Nutr.* 2018 Feb;57(1):1-24.

27 Thursby E, Juge N. Introduction to the human gut microbiota. *Biochem J.* 2017 Jun 1; 474(11): 1823–1836.

28 Zhu B, Wang X, Lanjuan L. Human gut microbiome: the second genome of human body. *Protein Cell.* 2010 Aug;1(8):718-25.

29 Tierney BT, Tan Y, Kostic AD, et al. Gene-level metagenomic architectures across diseases yield high-resolution microbiome diagnostic indicators. *Nature Comm.* 2021;12:2097.

30 Thursby E, Juge N. Introduction to the human gut microbiota. *Biochem J.* 2017 Jun 1; 474(11): 1823–1836.

31 Magne F, Gotteland M, Gauthier L, et al. The Firmicutes/Bacteroidetes Ratio: A Relevant Marker of Gut Dysbiosis in Obese Patients? *Nutrients.* 2020 May;12(5):1474.

32 Rutsch A, Kantsjo JB, Ronchi F. The Gut-Brain Axis: How Microbiota and Host Inflammasome Influence Brain Physiology and Pathology. *Front Immunol.* 2020 Dec 10;11:604179.

33 Lurie DI. An Integrative Approach to Neuroinflammation in Psychiatric disorders and Neuropathic Pain. *J Exp Neurosci.* 2018; 12: 1179069518793639.

34 Kwon HS, Koh SH. Neuroinflammation in neurodegenerative disorders: the roles of microglia and astrocytes. *Transl Neurodegener.* 2020 Nov 26;9(1):42.

35 Bested AC, Logan AC, Selhub EM. Intestinal microbiota, probiotics and mental health: from Metchnikoff to modern advances: part I - autointoxication revisited. *Gut Pathog.* 2013;5:5.

36 Guo S, Al-Sadi R, Said HM, et al. Lipopolysaccharide causes an increase in intestinal tight junction permeability in vitro and in vivo by inducing enterocyte membrane expression and localization of TLR-4 and CD14. *Am J Pathol.* 2013 Feb;182(2):375-87.

37 Seki E, Schnabl B. Role of innate immunity and the microbiota in liver fibrosis: crosstalk between the liver and gut. *J Physiol.* 2012;590(3):447–458.

38 Liu X, Yang W, Guan Z, et al. There are only four basic modes of cell death, although there are many ad-hoc variants adapted to different situations. *Cell Biosci.* 2018;6(2018).

[39] Cepelak I, Dodig S, Dodig DC. Ferroptosis: Regulated Cell Death. *Arh Hig Rada Toksikol.* 2020 Jun;71(2):99–109.

[40] Lai B, Wu CH, Wu CY, et al. Ferroptosis and Autoimmune Diseases. *Front Immunol.* 2022;13:916664.

[41] Lu J, Xu F, Lu H. LncRNA PVT1 regulates ferroptosis through miR-214-mediated TFR1 and p53. *Life Sci.* 2020;260:118305.

[42] Mayr L, Grabherr F, Schwärzler J, et al. Dietary lipids fuel GPX4-restricted enteritis resembling Crohn's disease. *Nat Commun.* 2020;11:1775.

[43] Xu M, Tao J, Yang Y, Tan S, et al. Ferroptosis involves in intestinal epithelial cell death in ulcerative colitis. *Cell Death Dis.* 2020;11:86.

[44] Mayr L, Grabherr F, Schwärzler J, et al. Dietary lipids fuel GPX4-restricted enteritis resembling Crohn's disease. *Nat Commun.* 2020;11:1775.

[45] Mayr L, Grabherr F, Schwärzler J, et al. Dietary lipids fuel GPX4-restricted enteritis resembling Crohn's disease. *Nat Commun.* 2020;11:1775.

[46] Deng F, Zhao BC, Yang X, et al. The gut microbiota metabolite capsiate promotes Gpx4 expression by activating TRPV1 to inhibit intestinal ischemia reperfusion-induced ferroptosis. *Gut Microbes.* 2021 Jan-Dec;13(1):1-21.

[47] Guan Z, Jin X, Guan Z, et al. The gut microbiota metabolite capsiate regulate SLC2A1 expression by targeting HIF-1α to inhibit knee osteoarthritis-induced ferroptosis. *Aging Cell.* 2023 Jun;22(6):e13807.

[48] Pyun BJ, Choi S, Lee Y, et al. Capsiate, a nonpungent capsaicin-like compound, inhibits angiogenesis and vascular permeability via a direct inhibition of Src kinase activity. *Cancer Res.* 2008 Jan 1;68(1):227-35.

[49] Zang Y, Fan L, Chen J, et al. Improvement of Lipid and Glucose Metabolism by Capsiate in Palmitic Acid-Treated HepG2 Cells via Activation of the AMPK/SIRT1 Signaling Pathway. *J Agric Food Chem.* 2018;66(26):6772–6781.

[50] Wang S, Liu W, Wang J, et al. Curculigoside inhibits ferroptosis in ulcerative colitis through the induction of GPX4. *Life Sci.* 2020;259:118356.

[51] Xu M, Tao J, Yang Y, et al. Ferroptosis involves in intestinal epithelial cell death in ulcerative colitis. *Cell Death Dis.* 2020;11:86.

[52] Barnabaei L, Laplantine E, Mbongo W, et al. NF-κB: At the Borders of Autoimmunity and Inflammation. *Front Immunol.* 2021;12:716469.

[53] Pashnina IA, Krivolapova IM, Fedotkina TV, et al. Antinuclear Autoantibodies in Health: Autoimmunity Is Not a Synonym of Autoimmune Disease. *Antibodies (Basel).* 2021 Mar;10(1):9.

[54] Shome M, Chung Y, Chavan R, et al. Serum autoantibodyome reveals that healthy individuals share common autoantibodies. *Cell Rep*orts. 2022;39(9):110873

[55] Nigrovic PA. The autoinflammatory diseases: An overview. Available at: https://www.uptodate.com/contents/the-autoinflammatory-diseases-an-overview#.

[56] Dominguex-Bello MG, Godoy-Vitorino F, Knight R, et al. Role of the microbiome in human development. *Gut.* 2019 Jun;68(6):1108–1114.

[57] Greenhalgh K, Meyer KM, Aagaard KM, et al. The human gut microbiome in health: establishment and resilience of microbiota over a lifetime. *Environ Microbiol.* 2016 Jul;18(7):2103-16.

[58] Guinane CM, Cotter PD. Role of the gut microbiota in health and chronic gastrointestinal disease: understanding a hidden metabolic organ. *Ther Adv Gastroenterol.* 2013;6:295–308

[59] Kahrstrom CT, Pariente N, Weiss U. Intestinal microbiota in health and disease. *Nature.* 2016;535:47.

[60] Clemente JC, Ursell LK, Parfrey LW, et al. The impact of the gut microbiota on human health: an integrative view. *Cell.* 2012;148:1258–1270.

[61] Takiishi T, Morales Fenero CI, Saraiva Camara NO, et al. Intestinal barrier and gut microbiota: Shaping our immune responses throughout life. *Tissue Barriers.* 2017;5(4):e1373208.

[62] Wei P, Keller C, Li L. Neuropeptides in gut-brain axis and their influence on host immunity and stress. *Comput Struct Biotechnol J.* 2020;18:843–851.

[63] Wang P, Liu YQ. Ferroptosis: A Critical Moderator in the Life Cycle of Immune Cells. *Front Immunol.* 2022 May 10;13:877634.

[64] Thursby E, Juge N. Introduction to the human gut microbiota. *Biochem J.* 2017 Jun 1;474(11):1823–1836.

[65] Singh RK, Chang HW, Yan D, et al. Influence of diet on the gut microbiome and implications for human health. *J Transl Med.* 2017 Apr 8;15(1):73.

[66] Albracht-Shulte K, Islam T, Johnson P, et al. Systematic Review of Beef Protein Effects on Gut Microbiota: Implications for Health. *Adv Nutr.* 2021 Feb 1;12(1):102-114.

[67] Wu S, Bhat ZF, Gounder RS, et al. Effect of Dietary Protein and Processing on Gut Microbiota—A Systematic Review. *Nutrients.* 2022 Feb;14(3):453.

[68] Mariotti F. Plant Protein, Animal Protein, and Protein Quality. Academic Press; Cambridge, MA, USA: 2017. Vegetarian and plant-based diets in health and disease prevention; pp. 621–642.

[69] Seal CJ, Courtin CM, Venema K, et al. Health benefits of whole grain: effects on dietary carbohydrate quality, the gut microbiome, and consequences of processing. *Compr Rev Food Sci Food Saf.* 2021 May;20(3):2742-2768.

[70] Fasano A. Intestinal Permeability and its Regulation by Zonulin: Diagnostic and Therapeutic Implications. *Clin Gastroenterol Hepatol.* 2012 Oct;10(10):1096–1100.

[71] Zhao GP, Li JW, Yang FW, et al. Nitrogen contaminants damage on intestinal epithelial tight junctions: a review. *Environ Chem Letters.* 2021;19:4549-61.

[72] Marino M, Mele E, Viggiano A, et al. Pleiotropic Outcomes of Glyphosate Exposure: From Organ Damage to Effects on Inflammation, Cancer, Reproduction and Development. *Int J Mol Sci.* 2021 Nov;22(22):12606.

[73] Fasano A. Intestinal Permeability and its Regulation by Zonulin: Diagnostic and Therapeutic Implications. *Clin Gastroenterol Hepatol.* 2012 Oct; 10(10): 1096–1100.

[74] Fasano A. All disease begins in the (leaky) gut: role of zonulin-mediated gut permeability in the pathogenesis of some chronic inflammatory diseases. *F1000Res.* 2020;9:F1000 Faculty Rev-69.

[75] Binienda A, Twardowska A, Makaro A, et al. Dietary Carbohydrates and Lipids in the Pathogenesis of Leaky Gut Syndrome: An Overview. *Int J Mol Sci.* 2020 Nov; 21(21): 8368.

[76] Paik DC, Wendel TD, Freeman HP. Cured meat consumption and hypertension: an analysis from NHANES III (1988-94). *Nutr Res.* 2005 Dec;25(12):1049-60.

[77] Micha R, Wallace SK, Mozaffarian D. Red and processed meat consumption and risk of incident coronary heart disease, stroke, and diabetes mellitus: a systematic review and meta-analysis. *Circulation.* 2010 Jun 1;121(21):2271-83.

[78] Gonzalez CA, Jekszyn P, Pera G, et al. Meat intake and risk of stomach and esophageal adenocarcinoma within the European Prospective Investigation Into Cancer and Nutrition (EPIC). *J Natl Cancer Inst.* 2006 Mar 1;98(5):345-54.

[79] Santarelli RL, Pierre F, Corpet DE. Processed meat and colorectal cancer: a review of epidemiologic and experimental evidence. *Nutr Cancer.* 2008;60(2):131-44.

[80] Jiang R, Paik DC, Hankinson JL, et al. Cured meat consumption, lung function, and chronic obstructive pulmonary disease among United States adults. *Am J Respir Crit Care Med.* 2007 Apr 15;175(8):798-804.

[81] U.S. National Library of Medicine. Polycyclic Aromatic Hydrocarbons: Evaluation of Sources and Effects. Appendix C: Human-Cancer Risk Assessment. Available at: https://www.ncbi.nlm.nih.gov/books/NBK217747/.

[82] Srour B, Kordahi MC, Bonazzi E, et al. Ultra-processed foods and human health: from epidemiological evidence to mechanistic insights. *The Lancet.* 2022 Dec;7(12):P1128-40.

[83] Shi Z. Gut Microbiota: An Important Link between Western Diet and Chronic Diseases. *Nutrients.* 2019 Oct;11(10):2287.

[84] Srour B, Touvier M. Ultra-processed foods and human health: What do we already know and what will further research tell us? eClinicalMed. 2021 Feb;32:100747.

[85] Rapin JR, Wiernsperger N. Possible Links between Intestinal Permeablity and Food Processing: A Potential Therapeutic Niche for Glutamine. *Clinics (Sao Paulo).* 2010 Jun; 65(6): 635–643.

[86] U.S. National Library of Medicine. Effect of advanced glycation end product intake on inflammation and aging: a systematic review. Available at: https://www.ncbi.nlm.nih.gov/books/NBK291556/.

[87] Reddy CP, Aryal P, Darkwah EK. Advanced Glycation End Products in Health and Disease. *Microorganisms.* 2022 Sep;10(9):1848.

[88] Phuong-Nguyen K, McNeill BA, Aston-Mourney K, et al. Advanced Glycation End-Products and Their Effects on Gut Health. *Nutrients.* 2023 Jan;15(2):405.

[89] Siljander H, Jason E, Ruohtula T, et al. Effect of Early Feeding on Intestinal Permeability and Inflammation Markers in Infants with Genetic Susceptibility to Type 1 Diabetes: A Randomized Clinical Trial. *J Pediatr.* 2021;238:305–311.e3.

[90] Seiquer I, Rubio LA, Peinado MJ, et al. Maillard reaction products modulate gut microbiota composition in adolescents. *Mol Nutr Food Res.* 2014;58:1552–1560.

[91] Phuong-Nguyen K, McNeill BA, Aston-Mourney K, et al. Advanced Glycation End-Products and Their Effects on Gut Health. *Nutrients.* 2023 Jan;15(2):405.

[92] Aoun A, Darwish F, Hamod N. The Influence of the Gut Microbiome on Obesity in Adults and the Role of Probiotics, Prebiotics, and Synbiotics for Weight Loss. *Prev Nutr Food Sci.* 2020 Jun 30;25(2):113–123.

[93] Inczefi O, Bascur P, Resal T, et al. The Influence of Nutrition on Intestinal Permeability and the Microbiome in Health and Disease. *Front Nutr.* 2022 Apr 25;9:2022.

[94] Murphy EA, Velazquez KT, Herbert KM. Influence of high-fat diet on gut microbiota: a driving force for chronic disease risk. *Curr Opin Clin Nutr Metab Care.* 2015 Sep;18(5):515-20.

[95] Rohr MW, Narasimhulu CA, Rudeski-Rohr T, et al. Negative Effects of a High-Fat Diet on Intestinal Permeability: A Review. *Adv Nutr.* 2020 Jan 1;11(1):77-91.

[96] Christ A, Lauterbacjh M, Latz E. Western Diet and the Immune System: An Inflammatory Connection. *Immunity*. 2019 Nov;51(5):794-811.

[97] Pipoyan D, Stepanyan St, Stepanyan Se, et al. The Effect of Trans Fatty Acids on Human Health: Regulation and Consumption Patterns. *Foods*. 2021 Oct;10(10):2452.

[98] Qi L. Fried Foods, Gut Microbiota, and Glucose Metabolism. *Diabetes Care*. 2021 Sep;44(9):1907–1909.

[99] Bode C, Bode JC. Effect of alcohol consumption on the gut. *Best Pract Res Clin Gastroenterol*. 2003 Aug;17(4):575-92.

[100] Engen PA, Green SJ, Voigt RM. The Gastrointestinal Microbiome: Alcohol Effects on the Composition of Intestinal Microbiota. *Alcohol Res*. 2015;37(2):223-36.

[101] Macdonald LE, Brett J, Kelton D, et al. A systematic review and meta-analysis of the effects of pasteurization on milk vitamins, and evidence for raw milk consumption and other health-related outcomes. *J Food Prot*. 2011 Nov;74(11):1814-32.

[102] The Weston A. Price Foundation. Ultra-Pasteurized Milk. Available at: https://www.westonaprice.org/health-topics/modern-foods/ultra-pasteurized-milk/#gsc.tab=0.

[103] Woodford KB. Casomorphins and Gliadorphins Have Diverse Systemic Effects Spanning Gut, Brain and Internal Organs. *Int J Environ Res Public Health*. 2021 Aug;18(15):7911.

[104] Vanhaecke T, Bretin O., Poirel M, et al. Drinking Water Source and Intake Are Associated with Distinct Gut Microbiota Signatures in US and UK Populations. *J Nutr*. 2022 Jan 11;152(1):171-182.

[105] National Academies of Sciences, Engineering, and Medicine. Report Sets Dietary Intake Levels for Water, Salt, and Potassium To Maintain Health and Reduce Chronic Disease Risk. Available at: https://www.nationalacademies.org/news/2004/02/report-sets-dietary-intake-levels-for-water-salt-and-potassium-to-maintain-health-and-reduce-chronic-disease-risk.

[106] McCarthy D, Dale M. The leucocytosis of exercise. *Sports Med*. 1988;6(6):333-363.

[107] Wolach B, Falk B, Gavrieli R, et al. Neutrophil function response to aerobic and anaerobic exercise in female judoka and untrained subjects. *Br J Sports Med*. 2000;34(1):23-28.

[108] Ortega E, Collazos ME, Maynar M, et al. Stimulation of the phagocytic function of neutrophils in sedentary men after acute moderate exercise. *Eur J Appl Physiol Occup Physiol*. 1993;66(1):60-64.

[109] Smith J, McKenzie S, Telford R, et al. Why does moderate exercise enhance, but intense training depress, immunity. *Behavior Immun*. 1992:155-168.

[110] Pedersen BK, Ullum H. NK cell response to physical activity: possible mechanisms of action. *Med Sci Sports Exerc*. 1994;26(2):140-146.

[111] Suzui M, Kawai T, Kimura H, et al. Natural killer cell lytic activity and CD56(dim) and CD56(bright) cell distributions during and after intensive training. *J Appl Physiol*. 1985;96(6):2167-2173.

[112] Timmons BW, Cieslak T. Human natural killer cell subsets and acute exercise: a brief review. *Exerc Immunol Rev*. 2008;14:8-23.

[113] Kinashi Y, Hase K. Partners in Leaky Gut Syndrome: Intestinal Dysbiosis and Autoimmunity. *Front Immunol*. 2021 Apr 22;12:673708.

[114] Köhling HL, Plummer SF, Marchesi JR, et al. The microbiota and autoimmunity: Their role in thyroid autoimmune diseases. *Clin Immunol*. 2017;183:63–74.

[115] Monda V, Villano I, Messina A, et al. Exercise Modifies the Gut Microbiota with Positive Health Effects. *Oxidative Med Cell Longevity*. 2017;217:3831972.

[116] Bressa C, Bailen-Andrino M, Perez-Santiago J, et al. Differences in gut microbiota profile between women with active lifestyle and sedentary women. *PLoS One*. 2017 Feb 10;12(2):e0171352.

[117] Clarke SF, Murphy EF, O'Sullivan O, et al. Exercise and associated dietary extremes impact on gut microbial diversity. *Gut*. 2014 Dec;63(12):1913-20.

[118] Bermon S, Petriz B, Kajeniene A, et al. The microbiota: an exercise immunology perspective. *Exerc Immunol Rev*. 2015;21:70-9.

[119] Chenard T, Prevost K, Dube J, et al. Immune System Modulations by Products of the Gut Microbiota. *Vaccines* (Basel). 2020 Sep; 8(3): 461.

[120] Leonel AJ, Alvarez-Leite JI. Butyrate: implications for intestinal function. *Curr Opin Clin Nutr Metab Care*. 2012 Sep;15(5):474-9.

[121] Estaki M, Pither J, Baumeister P, et al. Cardiorespiratory fitness as a predictor of intestinal microbial diversity and distinct metagenomic functions. *Microbiome*. 2016 Aug 8;4(1)42:

[122] Ringseis R, Eder K, Mooren FC, et al. Metabolic signals and innate immune activation in obesity and exercise. *Exerc Immunol Rev*. 2015;21:58-68.

[123] Soderholm JD, Perdue MH. Stress and intestinal barrier function. *Am J Physiol Gastrointest Liver Physiol*. 2001;280:G7-13.

[124] Geng S, Yang L, Cheng F, et al. Gut Microbiota Are Associated With Psychological Stress-Induced Defections in Intestinal and Blood–Brain Barriers. *Front Microbiol*. 2020 Jan 15;10:3067.

[125] Ogawa Y, Miyoshi C, Obana N, et al. Gut microbiota depletion by chronic antibiotic treatment alters the sleep/wake architecture and sleep EEG power spectra in mice. *Sci Reports*. 2020;10:19554.

[126] Smith RP, Easson C, Lyle SM, et al. Gut microbiome diversity is associated with sleep physiology in humans. *PLoS One*. 2019;14(10):e0222394.

[127] Garbarino S, Lanteri P, Bragazzi NL, et al. Role of sleep deprivation in immune-related disease risk and outcomes. *Commun Biol*. 2021;4:1304.

[128] Dhingra D, Michael M, Rajput H, et al. Dietary fibre in foods: a review. *J Food Sci Technol*. 2012 Jun;49(3):255–266.

[129] Miketinas DC, Bray GA, Beyl RA, et al. Fiber Intake Predicts Weight Loss and Dietary Adherence in Adults Consuming Calorie-Restricted Diets: The POUNDS Lost (Preventing Overweight Using Novel Dietary Strategies) Study. *J Nutr*. 2019 Oct 1;149(10):1742-1748.

[130] Arayici ME, Mert-Ozupek N, Yalcin F, et al. Soluble and Insoluble Dietary Fiber Consumption and Colorectal Cancer Risk: A Systematic Review and Meta-Analysis. *Nutr Cancer*. 2022;74(7):2412-2425.

[131] Lipsky H, Gloger M, Frishman WH. Dietary fiber for reducing blood cholesterol. *J Clin Pharmacol*. 1990;30(8):699-703.

[132] Marlett JA, Kajs TM, Fischer MH. An unfermented gel component of psyllium seed husk promotes laxation as a lubricant in humans. *Am J Clin Nutr*. 2000;72:784-9.

[133] Hanif palla A, Gilani AH. Dual effectiveness of flaxseed in constipation and diarrhea: Possible mechanism. *J Ethnopharmacol*. 2015;169:60-8.

[134] National Toxicology Program. Toxicology study of senna (CAS No. 8013-11-4) in C57BL/6NTAC mice and toxicology and carcinogenesis study of senna in genetically modified C3B6.129F1/Tac-Trp53tm1Brd haploinsufficient mice (feed studies). *Natl Toxicol Program Genet Modif Model Rep*. 2012;(15):1-114.

[135] Rao SSC, Brenner DM. Efficacy and Safety of Over-the-Counter Therapies for Chronic Constipation: An Updated Systematic Review. *Am J Gastroenterol*. 2021 Jun;116(6):1156–1181.

[136] Cirillo C, Capasso R. Constipation and Botanical Medicines: An Overview. *Phytother Res*. 2015;29:1488-93.

[137] Sears ME. Chelation: Harnessing and Enhancing Heavy Metal Detoxification—A Review. *ScientificWorldJournal*. 2013; 2013: 219840.

[138] Surai PF. Silymarin as a Natural Antioxidant: An Overview of the Current Evidence and Perspectives. *Antioxidants (Basel)*. 2015 Mar;4(1):204–247.

[139] Jalali M, Mahmoodi M, Mosallazezhad Z, et al. The effects of curcumin supplementation on liver function, metabolic profile and body composition in patients with non-alcoholic fatty liver disease: A systematic review and meta-analysis of randomized controlled trials. *Complement Ther Med*. 2020 Jan;48:102283.

[140] Hodges RE, Minich DM. Modulation of Metabolic Detoxification Pathways Using Foods and Food-Derived Components: A Scientific Review with Clinical Application. *J Nutr Metab*. 2015;2015:760689.

[141] Ghareghomi S, Rahban M, Moosavi-Movahedi Z, et al. The Potential Role of Curcumin in Modulating the Master Antioxidant Pathway in Diabetic Hypoxia-Induced Complications. *Molecules*. 2021 Dec;26(24):7658.

[142] Hodges RE, Minich DM. Modulation of Metabolic Detoxification Pathways Using Foods and Food-Derived Components: A Scientific Review with Clinical Application. *J Nutr Metab*. 2015;2015:760689.

[143] Colak E, Ustuner MC, Tekin N, et al. The hepatocurative effects of Cynara scolymus L. leaf extract on carbon tetrachloride-induced oxidative stress and hepatic injury in rats. *Springerplus*. 2016;5:216.

[144] Yarnell E. Botanical medicines for the urinary tract. *World J Urol*. 2002;20(5):285–293.

[145] Clare BA, Conroy RS, Spelman K. The diuretic effect in human subjects of an extract of Taraxacum officinale folium over a single day. *J Altern Complement Med*. 2009 Aug;15(8):929-34.

[146] Esra AS, Betul AY. Effect of Taraxacum officinale L. ethanol extract against kidney injuries induced by paracetamol in rats. *GSC Biol Pharm Sci*. 2022;21(01):144-151.

[147] Ren YS, Zheng Y, Duan H, et al. Dandelion polyphenols protect against acetaminophen-induced hepatotoxicity in mice via activation of the Nrf-2/HO-1 pathway and inhibition of the JNK signaling pathway. *Chin J Nat Med*. 2020 Feb;18(2):103-113.

[148] Patangia DV, Ryan CA, Dempsey E, et al. Impact of antibiotics on the human microbiome and consequences for host health. *Microbiologyopen*. 2022 Feb;11(1):e1260.

[149] Zaura E, Brandt BW, de Mattos MJT, et al. Same Exposure but Two Radically Different Responses to Antibiotics: Resilience of the Salivary Microbiome versus Long-Term Microbial Shifts in Feces. *mBio.* 2015 Nov 10;6(6):e01693-15.

[150] Feng Y, Huang Y, Wang Y, et al. Antibiotics induced intestinal tight junction barrier dysfunction is associated with microbiota dysbiosis, activated NLRP3 inflammasome and autophagy. *PLoS One.* 2019 Jun 18;14(6):e0218384.

[151] Hung IY, Parathan P, Boonma P, et al. Antibiotic exposure postweaning disrupts the neurochemistry and function of enteric neurons mediating colonic motor activity. *Am J Physiol Gastrointest Liver Physiol.* 2020 Jun 1;318(6):G1042–G1053.

[152] Bjarnason I, Takeuchi K. Intestinal permeability in the pathogenesis of NSAID-induced enteropathy. *J Gastroenterol.* 2009;44 Suppl 19:23-9.

[153] Sigthorsson G, Tibble J, Hayllar J, et al. Intestinal permeability and inflammation in patients on NSAIDs. *Gut.* 1998 Oct;43(4):506-11.

[154] Wang X, Tang Q, Hou H, et al. Gut Microbiota in NSAID Enteropathy: New Insights From Inside. *Front Cell Infect Microbiol.* 2021;11:679396.

[155] Rogers MAM, Aronoff DM. The Influence of Nonsteroidal Anti-Inflammatory Drugs on the Gut Microbiome. *Clin Microbiol Infect.* 2016 Feb;22(2):178.e1–178.e9.

[156] Foslund SK, Chakaroun R, Zimmermann-Kogadeeva M, et al. Combinatorial, additive and dose-dependent drug–microbiome associations. *Nature.* 2021;600:500-505.

[157] Vila AV, Collij V, Sanna S, et al. Impact of commonly used drugs on the composition and metabolic function of the gut microbiota. *Nat Commun.* 2020 Jan 17;11(1):362.

[158] Forslund K, Hildebrand F, Nielsen T, et al. Disentangling type 2 diabetes and metformin treatment signatures in the human gut microbiota. *Nature.* 2015;528:262–6.

[159] Weersma RK, Zhernakova A, Fu J. Interaction between drugs and the gut microbiome. *Gut.* 2020 Aug;69(8):1510–1519.

[160] Galdeano CM, Cazorla SI, Dumit JML, et al. Beneficial Effects of Probiotic Consumption on the Immune System. *Ann Nutr Metab.* 2019;74(2):115-124.

[161] De LeBlanc ADM, Dogi CA, Galdeano CM, et al. Effect of the administration of a fermented milk containing Lactobacillus casei DN-114001 on intestinal microbiota and gut associated immune cells of nursing mice and after weaning until immune maturity. *BMC Immunol.* 2008 Jun 13;9:27.

[162] Pandrey KR, Naik SR, Vakil BV. Probiotics, prebiotics and synbiotics- a review. *J Food Sci Technol.* 2015 Dec;52(12):7577–7587.

[163] Bell V, Ferraro J, Pimentel L, et al. One Health, Fermented Foods, and Gut Microbiota. *Foods.* 2018 Dec;7(12):195.

[164] Myhrstad MCW, Tunsjo H, Charnock C, et al. Dietary Fiber, Gut Microbiota, and Metabolic Regulation—Current Status in Human Randomized Trials. *Nutrients.* 2020 Mar;12(3):859.

[165] Bell V, Ferraro J, Pimentel L, et al. One Health, Fermented Foods, and Gut Microbiota. *Foods.* 2018 Dec;7(12):195.

[166] Vanasse A, Demers M, Hemiari A, et al. Obesity in Canada: where and how many? *Int J Obes.* 2006;30:677–683.

[167] Foster JA, Rinaman L, Cryan JF. Stress & the gut-brain axis: Regulation by the microbiome. *Neurobiol Stress.* 2017 Dec;7:124–136.

[168] Gronroos M, Parajuli A, Laitinen OH, et al. Short-term direct contact with soil and plant materials leads to an immediate increase in diversity of skin microbiota. *Microbiologyopen.* 2019 Mar;8(3):e00645.

[169] Lowry CA, Hollis JH, de Vires A, et al. Identification of an immune-responsive mesolimbocortical serotonergic system: Potential role in regulation of emotional behavior. *Neurosci.* 2007 May;146(2):756–72.

[170] Zhang S, Chen DC. Facing a new challenge: the adverse effects of antibiotics on gut microbiota and host immunity. *Chin Med J (Engl).* 2019 May 20;132(10):1135–1138.

[171] Niedzielin K, Kordecki H, Birkenfeld B. A controlled, double-blind, randomized study on the efficacy of Lactobacillus plantarum 299V in patients with irritable bowel syndrome. *Eur J Gastroenterol Hepatol.* 2001 Oct;13(10):1143-7.

[172] Ligaarden SC, Axelsson L, Naterstad K, et al. A candidate probiotic with unfavourable effects in subjects with irritable bowel syndrome: a randomised controlled trial. *BMC Gastroenterol.* 2010;10:16.

[173] Liu Y, Alookaran JJ, Rhoads JM. Probiotics in Autoimmune and Inflammatory Disorders. *Nutrients.* 2018 Oct;10(10):1537.

[174] Luca FD, Shoenfield Y. The microbiome in autoimmune diseases. *Clin Exp Immunol.* 2019 Jan;195(1):74–85.

[175] De Kivit S, Tobin MC, Forsyth CB, et al. Regulation of intestinal immune responses through TLR activation: implications for pro- and prebiotics. *Front Immunol.* 2014 Feb 18;5:60.

[176] Ku S, Park MS, Ji GE, et al. Review on Bifidobacterium bifidum BGN4: Functionality and Nutraceutical Applications as a Probiotic Microorganism. *Int J Mol Sci.* 2016 Sep 14;17(9):1544.

[177] Laparra JM, Olivares M, Gallina O, et al. Bifidobacterium longum CECT 7347 modulates immune responses in a gliadin-induced enteropathy animal model. *PLoS One.* 2012;7(2):e30744.

[178] Laparra JM, Sanz Y. Bifidobacteria inhibit the inflammatory response induced by gliadins in intestinal epithelial cells via modifications of toxic peptide generation during digestion. *J Cell Biochem.* 2010;109(4):801-807.

[179] Olivares M, Laparra M, Sanz Y. Oral administration of Bifidobacterium longum CECT 7347 modulates jejunal proteome in an in vivo gliadin-induced enteropathy animal model. *J Proteomics.* 2012;77:310-320.

[180] Olivares M, Castillejo G, Varea V, et al. Double-blind, randomised, placebo-controlled intervention trial to evaluate the effects of Bifidobacterium longum CECT 7347 in children with newly diagnosed coeliac disease. *Br J Nutr.* 2014 Jul 14;112(1):30-40.

[181] Klemenak M, Dolinšek J, Langerholc T, et al. Mičetić-Turk, D. Administration of bifidobacterium breve decreases the production of TNF-α in children with celiac disease. *Dig Dis Sci.* 2015;60(11):3386-3392.

[182] Vaghef-Mehrabany E, Aliour B, Homayouni-Rad A, et al. Probiotic supplementation improves inflammatory status in patients with rheumatoid arthritis. *Nutrition.* 2014 Apr;30(4):430-5.

[183] Calcinaro F, Dionisi S, Marinaro M, et al. Oral probiotic administration induces interleukin-10 production and prevents spontaneous autoimmune diabetes in the non-obese diabetic mouse. *Diabetologia.* 2005;48(8):1565-1575.

[184] Cheng FS, Pan D, Chang B, et al. Probiotic mixture VSL#3: An overview of basic and clinical studies in chronic diseases. *World J Clin Cases.* 2020 Apr 26;8(8):1361–1384.

[185] Batu ED, Akca UK, Basaran O, et al. Probiotic use in the prophylaxis of periodic fever, aphthous stomatitis, pharyngitis, and adenitis (PFAPA) syndrome: a retrospective cohort study. *Rheumatol Int.* 2022 Jul;42(7):1207-1211.

[186] Kullisaar T, Songisepp E, Aunapuu M, et al. Complete glutathione system in probiotic Lactobacillus fermentum ME-3. *Prikl Biokhim Mikrobiol.* 2010 Sep-Oct;46(5):527-31.

[187] Wang B, Wu G, Zhou Z, et al. Glutamine and intestinal barrier function. *Amino Acids.* 2015 Oct;47(10):2143-54.

[188] Shu XL, Yu TT, Kang K, et al. Effects of glutamine on markers of intestinal inflammatory response and mucosal permeability in abdominal surgery patients: A meta-analysis. *Exp Ther Med.* 2016 Dec;12(6):3499-3506.

[189] Kim MH, Kim H. The Roles of Glutamine in the Intestine and Its Implication in Intestinal Diseases. *Int J Mol Sci.* 2017 May;18(5):1051.

[190] Achamrah N, Dechelotte P, Coeffier M. Glutamine and the regulation of intestinal permeability: from bench to bedside. *Curr Opin Clin Nutr Metab Care.* 2017 Jan;20(1):86-91.

[191] Zhou Q, Verne ML, Fields JZ, et al. Randomised placebo-controlled trial of dietary glutamine supplements for postinfectious irritable bowel syndrome. *Gut.* 2019 Jun;68(6):996-1002.

[192] Godhia ML, Patel N. Colostrum - Its Composition, Benefits As A Nutraceutical : A Review. *Curr Res Nutr Food Sci.* 2013;1(1):34-37.

[193] Stewart MG. New insight into mode of action of ColostrininTM. *J Nutr Health Aging.* 2010;14:336.

[194] Boldogh I, Aguilera-Aguirre L, Bacsi A, et al. Colostrinin decreases hypersensitivity and allergic responses to common allergens. *Int Arch Allergy Immunol.* 2008;146(4):298–306.

[195] Halasa M, Maciejewska D, Baskiewicz-Halasa M, et al. Oral Supplementation with Bovine Colostrum Decreases Intestinal Permeability and Stool Concentrations of Zonulin in Athletes. *Nutrients.* 2017 Apr;9(4):370.

[196] Marchbank T, Davison G, Oakes JR, et al. The nutriceutical [SIC] bovine colostrum truncates the increase in gut permeability caused by heavy exercise in athletes. *Am J Physiol Gastrointest Liver Physiol.* 2011 Mar;300(3):G477-84.

[197] Playford RJ, MacDonald CE, Calnan DP, et al. Co-administration of the health food supplement, bovine colostrum, reduces the acute non-steroidal anti-inflammatory drug-induced increase in intestinal permeability. *Clin Sci (Lond).* 2001 Jun;100(6):627-33.

[198] Hung LH, Wu CH, Lin BF, et al. Hyperimmune colostrum alleviates rheumatoid arthritis in a collagen-induced arthritis murine model. *J Dairy Sci.* 2018 May;101(5):3778-3787.

[199] Sanctuary MR, Kain JN, Chen SY, et al. Pilot study of probiotic/colostrum supplementation on gut function in children with autism and gastrointestinal symptoms. *PLoS One*. 2019;14(1):e0210064.

[200] Pearce FL, Befus AD, Bienstock J. Mucosal mast cells. III. Effect of quercetin and other flavonoids on antigen-induced histamine secretion from rat intestinal mast cells. *J Allergy Clin Immunol*. 1984 Jun;73(6):819-23.

[201] Weng Z, Zhang B, Asadi S, et al. Quercetin is more effective than cromolyn in blocking human mast cell cytokine release and inhibits contact dermatitis and photosensitivity in humans. *PLoS One*. 2012;7(3):e33805.

[202] Gao W, Zan Y, Wang ZJ, et al. Quercetin ameliorates paclitaxel-induced neuropathic pain by stabilizing mast cells, and subsequently blocking PKCε-dependent activation of TRPV1. *Acta Pharmacol Sin*. 2016 Sep;37(9):1166-77.

[203] Penissi AB, Rudolph MI, Piezzi RS. Role of mast cells in gastrointestinal mucosal defense. *Biocell*. 2003 Aug;27(2):163-72.

[204] Shi T, Bian X, Yao Z, et al. Quercetin improves gut dysbiosis in antibiotic-treated mice. *Food Funct*. 2020 Sep 23;11(9):8003-8013.

[205] Shigeshiro M, Tanabe S, Suzuki T. Dietary polyphenols modulate intestinal barrier defects and inflammation in a murine model of colitis. *J Funct Foods*. 2013 Apr;5(2):949-55.

[206] de Medina FS, Calvez J, Romero JA, et al. Effect of quercitrin on acute and chronic experimental colitis in the rat. *J Pharmacol Experiment Ther*. 1996;278(2):771-9.

[207] Suzuki T, Hara H. Quercetin enhances intestinal barrier function through the assembly of zonula [corrected] occludens-2, occludin, and claudin-1 and the expression of claudin-4 in Caco-2 cells. *J Nutr*. 2009 May;139(5):965-74.

[208] Amasheh M, Schlichter S, Amasheh S, et al. Quercetin enhances epithelial barrier function and increases claudin-4 expression in Caco-2 cells. *J Nutr*. 2008 Jun;138(6):1067-73.

[209] D'Adamo P. Larch arabinogalactan. *J Naturopath Med*. 1996;6:33-37.

[210] Dion C, Chappuis E, Ripoll C. Does larch arabinogalactan enhance immune function? A review of mechanistic and clinical trials. *Nutr Metab (Lond)*. 2016;13:28.

[211] Daguet D, Pinheiro I, Verhelst A, et al. Arabinogalactan and fructooligosaccharides improve the gut barrier function in distinct areas of the colon in the Simulator of the Human Intestinal Microbial Ecosystem. *J Functional Foods*. 2016 Jan;20:369–379.

[212] Chen O, Sudakaran S, Blonquist T, et al. Effect of arabinogalactan on the gut microbiome: A randomized, double-blind, placebo-controlled, crossover trial in healthy adults. *Nutrition*. 2021 Oct;90:111273.

[213] Hagmar B, Ryd W, Skomedal H. Arabinogalactan blockade of experimental metastases to liver by murine hepatoma. *Invasion Metastasis*. 1991;11:348-355.

[214] Kelly GS. Larch arabinogalactan: clinical relevance of a novel immune-enhancing polysaccharide. *Altern Med Rev*. 1999 Apr;4(2):96-103.

[215] Dion C, Chappuis E, Ripoll C. Does larch arabinogalactan enhance immune function? A review of mechanistic and clinical trials. *Nutr Metab (Lond)*. 2016;13:28.

[216] Varani J, Dame MK, Rittie L, et al. Decreased Collagen Production in Chronologically Aged Skin. *Am J Pathol.* 2006 Jun;168(6):1861–1868.

[217] Graham MF, Diegelmann RF, Elson CO, et al. Collagen Content and Types in the Intestinal Strictures of Crohn's Disease. *Gastroenterology*, 1988;94:257-65.

[218] Chang WK, Yang KD, Shaio MF. Effect of glutamine on Th1 and Th2 cytokine responses of human peripheral blood mononuclear cells. *Clin Immunol.* 1999 Dec;93(3):294-301.

[219] Rao R, Samak G. Role of Glutamine in Protection of Intestinal Epithelial Tight Junctions. *J Epithel Biol Pharmacol.* 2012 Jan;5(Suppl 1-M7):47–54.

[220] Graham MF, Drucker DE, Diegelmann RF, et al. Collagen synthesis by human intestinal smooth muscle cells in culture. *Gastroenterology.* 1987 Feb 1;92(2):400-5.

[221] Chen Q, Chen O, Martins IM, et al. Collagen peptides ameliorate intestinal epithelial barrier dysfunction in immunostimulatory Caco-2 cell monolayers via enhancing tight junctions. *Food Funct.* 2017 Mar 22;8(3):1144-1151.

[222] Chevalier NR, Gazquez E, Bidault L, et al. How tissue mechanical properties affect enteric neural crest cell migration. *Sci Rep.* 2016 Feb 18;6:20927.

[223] Abrahams M, O'Grady R, Prawitt J. Effect of a Daily Collagen Peptide Supplement on Digestive Symptoms in Healthy Women: 2-Phase Mixed Methods Study. *JMIR Form Res.* 2022 May;6(5):e36339.

[224] Van Marle J, Aarsen PN, Lind A, et al. Deglycyrrhizinised liquorice (DGL) and the renewal of rat stomach epithelium. *Eur J Pharmacol.* 1981;72:219–225.

[225] Goso Y, Ogata Y, Ishihara K, et al. Effects of traditional herbal medicine on gastric mucin against ethanol-induced gastric injury in rats. *Comp Biochem Physiol C Pharmacol Toxicol Endocrinol.* 1996;113:17–21.

[226] Peterson CT, Sharma V, Uchitel S, et al. Prebiotic Potential of Herbal Medicines Used in Digestive Health and Disease. *J Altern Complement Med.* 2018 Jul;24(7):656-665.

[227] Setright R. Prevention of symptoms of gastric irritation (GERD) using two herbal formulas: An observational study. *J Australian Traditional-Med Soc.* 2017 Jun 1; 23(2):68–71.

[228] Peterson CT, Sharma V, Uchitel S, et al. Prebiotic Potential of Herbal Medicines Used in Digestive Health and Disease. *J Alternat Complement Med.* 2018 Jul 1;24(7):656–665.

[229] Watts CR, Rousseau B. Slippery elm, its biochemistry, and use as a complementary and alternative treatment for laryngeal irritation. *J Investigational Biochem.* 2012;1(1):17–23.

[230] Phan THL, Park SY, Jung HJ, et al. The Role of Processed Aloe vera Gel in Intestinal Tight Junction: An In Vivo and In Vitro Study. *Int J Mol Sci.* 2021 Jun 17;22(12):6515.

[231] Yu Y, Yan Y, Niu F, et al. Ferroptosis: a cell death connecting oxidative stress, inflammation and cardiovascular diseases. *Cell Death Discov.* 2021 Jul 26;7(1):193.

[232] Li Z, Liao X, Hu Y, et al. SLC27A4-mediated selective uptake of mono-unsaturated fatty acids promotes ferroptosis defense in hepatocellular carcinoma. *Free Radic Biol Med.* 2023;201:41-54.

[233] Lai B, Wu CH, Wu CY, et al. Ferroptosis and Autoimmune Diseases. *Front Immunol.* 2022;13:916664.

[234] Smallwood MJ, Nissim A, Knight AR, et al. Oxidative stress in autoimmune rheumatic diseases. *Free Radic Biol Med.* 2018 Sep;125:3-14.

[235] Savic S, Dickie LJ, Wittmann M, et al. Autoinflammatory syndromes and cellular responses to stress: pathophysiology, diagnosis and new treatment perspectives. *Best Pract Res Clin Rheumatol.* 2012 Aug;26(4):505-33.

[236] Perricone C, de Carolis C, Perricone R. Glutathione: a key player in autoimmunity. *Autoimmun Rev.* 2009 Jul;8(8):697-701.

[237] Yang KT, Chao TH, Wang IC, et al. Berberine protects cardiac cells against ferroptosis. *Tzu Chi Med J.* 2022;34(3):310-317.

[238] Ma H, Wang X, Zhang W, et al. Melatonin suppresses ferroptosis induced by high glucose via activation of the Nrf2/HO-1 signaling pathway in type 2 diabetic osteoporosis. *Oxid Med Cell Longev.* 2020;2020:9067610.

[239] Wang L, Wang C, Li X, et al. Melatonin and erastin emerge synergistic anti-tumor effects on oral squamous cell carcinoma by inducing apoptosis, ferroptosis, and inhibiting autophagy through promoting ROS. *Cell Mol Biol Lett.* 2023;28(1):36.

[240] Won JP, Kim E, Hur J, Lee HG, Lee WJ, Seo HG. Red clover (Trifolium pratense L.) extract inhibits ferroptotic cell death by modulating cellular iron homeostasis. *J Ethnopharmacol.* 2023;308:116267.

[241] Feng Q, Yang Y, Qiao Y, et al. Quercetin ameliorates diabetic kidney injury by inhibiting ferroptosis via activating Nrf2/HO-1 signaling pathway. *Am J Chin Med.* 2023;1-22.

[242] Abbasifard M, Khorramdelazad H, Rostamian A, et al. Effects of N-acetylcysteine on systemic lupus erythematosus disease activity and its associated complications: a randomized double-blind clinical trial study. *Trials.* 2023;24(1):129.

[243] Flora SD, Grassi C, Carati L. Attenuation of influenza-like symptomatology and improvement of cell-mediated immunity with long-term N-acetylcysteine treatment. *Eur Respiratory J.* 1997;10(7):1535–1541.

[244] Abbasifard M, Khorramdelazad H, Rostamian A, et al. Effects of N-acetylcysteine on systemic lupus erythematosus disease activity and its associated complications: a randomized double-blind clinical trial study. *Trials.* 2023;24(1):129.

[245] Shukla PK, Gangwar R, Manda B, et al. Rapid disruption of intestinal epithelial tight junction and barrier dysfunction by ionizing radiation in mouse colon in vivo: protection by N-acetyl-l-cysteine. *Am J Physiol Gastrointest Liver Physiol.* 2016 May 1;310(9):G705–G715.

[246] Chu M, Zhang MB, Liu YC, et al. Role of Berberine in the Treatment of Methicillin-Resistant Staphylococcus aureus Infections. *Sci Rep.* 2016; 6: 24748.

[247] Zou K, Li Z, Zhang U, et al. Advances in the study of berberine and its derivatives: a focus on anti-inflammatory and anti-tumor effects in the digestive system. *Acta Pharmacol Sin.* 2017 Feb;38(2):157-167.

[248] Tabeshpour J, Imenshahidi M, Hosseinzadeh H. A review of the effects of Berberis vulgaris and its major component, berberine, in metabolic syndrome. *Iran J Basic Med Sci.* 2017 May;20(5):557–568.

[249] Lan J, Zhao Y, Dong F, et al. Meta-analysis of the effect and safety of berberine in the treatment of type 2 diabetes mellitus, hyperlipemia and hypertension. *J Ehtnopharmacol*. 2015 Feb;161:69–81.

[250] Liang Y, Xu X, Yin M, et al. Effects of berberine on blood glucose in patients with type 2 diabetes mellitus: a systematic literature review and a meta-analysis. *Endocr J*. 2019 Jan 28;66(1):51-63.

[251] Habtemariam S. Berberine pharmacology and the gut microbiota: A hidden therapeutic link. *Pharm Res*. 2020 May;155:104722.

[252] Zhang X, Zhao Y, Xu J, et al. Modulation of gut microbiota by berberine and metformin during the treatment of high-fat diet-induced obesity in rats. *Sci Reports*. 2016 Sep 23;5:14405.

[253] Shen P, Jiao Y, Miao L, et al. Immunomodulatory effects of berberine on the inflamed joint reveal new therapeutic targets for rheumatoid arthritis management. *J Cell Mol Med*. 2020 Nov;24(21):12234–12245.

[254] Ehteshamfar SM, Akhbari M, Afshari JT, et al. Anti-inflammatory and immune-modulatory impacts of berberine on activation of autoreactive T cells in autoimmune inflammation. *J Cell Mol Med*. 2020 Dec;24(23):13573–13588.

[255] Bao L, Jin Y, Han J, et al. Berberine Regulates GPX4 to Inhibit Ferroptosis of Islet β Cells. *Planta Med*. 2023 Mar;89(3):254-261.

[256] Yang KT, Chao TH, Wang IC, et al. Berberine protects cardiac cells against ferroptosis. *Tzu Chi Med J*. 2022;34(3):310-317.

[257] Yu Y, Liu L, Wang X, et al. Modulation of glucagon-like peptide-1 release by berberine: in vivo and in vitro studies. *Biochem Pharmacol*. 2010 Apr 1;79(7):1000-6.

[258] Yue X, Liang J, Gu F, et al. Berberine activates bitter taste responses of enteroendocrine STC-1 cells. *Mol Cell Biochem*. 2018 Oct;447(1-2):21-32.

[259] Andersen A, Lund A, Knop FK, et al. Glucagon-like peptide 1 in health and disease. *Nat Rev Endocrinol*. 2018 Jul;14(7):390-403.

[260] Sun Y, Jin C, Zhang X, et al. Restoration of GLP-1 secretion by Berberine is associated with protection of colon enterocytes from mitochondrial overheating in diet-induced obese mice. *Nutr Diabetes*. 2018;8:53.

[261] Blais JE, Huang X, Zhao JV. Overall and Sex-Specific Effect of Berberine for the Treatment of Dyslipidemia in Adults: A Systematic Review and Meta-Analysis of Randomized Placebo-Controlled Trials. *Drugs*. 2023 Apr;83(5):403-427.

[262] Blais JE, Huang X, Zhao JV. Overall and Sex-Specific Effect of Berberine for the Treatment of Dyslipidemia in Adults: A Systematic Review and Meta-Analysis of Randomized Placebo-Controlled Trials. *Drugs*. 2023 Apr;83(5):403-427.

[263] Zhao JV, Yeung WF, Chan YH, et al. Effect of Berberine on Cardiovascular Disease Risk Factors: A Mechanistic Randomized Controlled Trial. *Nutrients*. 2021;13(8).

[264] Li Y, Ma H, Zhang Y, et al. Effect of berberine on insulin resistance in women with polycystic ovary syndrome: study protocol for a randomized multicenter controlled trial. *Trials*. 2013;14:226.

[265] An Y, Sun Z, Zhang Y, et al. The use of berberine for women with polycystic ovary syndrome undergoing IVF treatment. *Clin Endocrinol (Oxf)*. 2014 Mar;80(3):425-31.

[266] Wei W, Zhao H, Wang A, et al. A clinical study on the short-term effect of berberine in comparison to metformin on the metabolic characteristics of women with polycystic ovary syndrome. *Eur J Endocrinol.* 2012 Jan;166(1):99-105.

[267] Sánchez-Quintero MJ, Delgado J, et al. Beneficial Effects of Essential Oils from the Mediterranean Diet on Gut Microbiota and Their Metabolites in Ischemic Heart Disease and Type-2 Diabetes Mellitus. *Nutrients.* 2022 Nov 3;14(21):4650.

[268] Di Vito M, Bellardi MG, Sanguinetti M, et al. Potent In Vitro Activity of Citrus aurantium Essential Oil and Vitis vinifera Hydrolate Against Gut Yeast Isolates From Irritable Bowel Syndrome Patients-The Right Mix for Potential Therapeutic Use. *Nutrients.* 2020 May 7;12(5):E1329.

[269] Wang L, Zhang Y, Fan G, et al. Effects of orange essential oil on intestinal microflora in mice. *J Sci Food Agric.* 2019 Jun;99(8):4019-4028.

[270] Qu SS, Zhang Y, Ren JN, et al. Effect of different ways of ingesting orange essential oil on blood immune index and intestinal microflora in mice. *J Sci Food Agric.* 2023 Jan 15;103(1):380-388.

[271] Leong W, Huang G, Khan I, et al. Patchouli Essential Oil and Its Derived Compounds Revealed Prebiotic-Like Effects in C57BL/6J Mice. *Front Pharmacol.* 2019 Oct 17;10:1229.

[272] Thapa S, Luna RA, Chumpitazi BP, et al. Peppermint oil effects on the gut microbiome in children with functional abdominal pain. *Clin Transl Sci.* 2022 Jan 20. Online ahead of print.

[273] Wan L, Li Y, Zhang Z, et al. Methylenetetrahydrofolate reductase and psychiatric diseases. *Transl Psychiatry.* 2018;8:242.

[274] Rainero I, Vacca A, Roveta F, et al. Targeting MTHFR for the treatment of migraines. *Expert Opin Ther Targets.* 2019 Jan;23(1):29-37.

[275] Chita DS, Tudor A, Christodorescu R, et al. MTHFR Gene Polymorphisms Prevalence and Cardiovascular Risk Factors Involved in Cardioembolic Stroke Type and Severity. *Brain Sci.* 2020 Jul 24;10(8):476.

[276] Zhang L, Chen B. Correlation between MTHFR polymorphisms and glaucoma: A meta-analysis. *Mol Genet Genomic Med.* 2019 Apr;7(4):e00538.

[277] Kim YI. Role of the MTHFR polymorphisms in cancer risk modification and treatment. *Future Oncol.* 2009 May;5(4):523-42.

[278] Wilcken B, Bamforth F, Li Z, et al. Geographical and ethnic variation of the 677C>T allele of 5,10 methylenetetrahydrofolate reductase (MTHFR): findings from over 7000 newborns from 16 areas world wide. *J Med Genetics.* 2003;40(8):619–25.

[279] Schneider JA, Rees DC, Liu YT, et al. Worldwide distribution of a common methylenetetrahydrofolate reductase mutation. *Am J Human Genetics.* 1998;62(5):1258–60.

[280] Ge Q, Gu X, Yu W, et al. Antinuclear antibodies in healthy population: Positive association with abnormal tissue metabolism, inflammation and immune dysfunction. *Int Immunopharmacol.* 2022 Dec;113(Pt A):109292.

[281] Pahnina IA, Krivolapova IM, Fedotkina TV, et al. Antinuclear Autoantibodies in Health: Autoimmunity Is Not a Synonym of Autoimmune Disease. *Antibodies (Basel).* 2021 Mar;10(1):9.

INDEX

N

N-Acetyl cysteine (NAC), 91-94, 101, 103
N-nitroso compounds, 45
necrosis, 18
neurological disorders/conditions, 8, 11, 13, 69
neuropeptides, 38
nonalcoholic fatty liver disease, 13
non-Hodgkin lymphoma, 37
nonessential amino acids, 87, 88
nonself-particles, 32
nutrigenomics, 42, 43
nutrition, 41-48, 78, 93

O

obesity, 11, 13, 20, 46, 52, 78, 79, 94
oregano essential oil, 63, 64, 65, 66

P

packaged goods, 45
Paneth cells, 17
Parkinson's disease, 8, 13
peppermint essential oil, 63, 64, 65, 66
pepsin, 15, 16, 32
phages, 63, 64, 65, 66, 67
physical activity, 11, 49-52
placenta, 10, 24, 87
plasma cells, 23, 24, 25, 27, 37
polyunsaturated fatty acids, 19, 44, 92
probiotics, 11, 43, 46, 58, 76-82, 84, 102
processed meats, 44-45
proctoscopy, 108
proline, 83, 86, 87, 88, 104
propionate, 8, 52, 86, 89
prostaglandins, 17, 36

prunes/prune juice, 60
psyllium, 59, 60

Q

quercetin, 85, 93, 102, 104

R

reactive oxygen species, 19, 29, 91, 92, 94
rheumatic factor, 109
rhinitis, 37

S

S-adenosyl methionine, 98
second brain, 8, 74
self-particles, 32, 33
senescence, 17, 18, 45
senna, 61, 62
secretin, 16
serotonin, 8, 30, 52, 54, 98
short-chain fatty acids, 8, 51, 52, 74, 86, 95, 96
sigmoidoscopy, 107
sleep, 11, 31, 53, 54, 100, 102, 103
slippery elm bark, 90-91, 103
stimulant herbal laxatives, 59, 61-62
stool DNA test, 106
stress, 8, 11, 53, 78, 79, 88, 99, 102
sugar, 43, 45, 46, 47, 48, 66, 77, 78, 97, 106, 110
synbiotics, 11, 76-82
synthetic drugs, 73-74

T

T cells, 15, 23, 24, 25, 26, 27, 33, 35, 36, 50, 77
telomeres, 18, 45
Th1, 30, 35, 50, 51
Th2, 30, 35, 50, 51
Th17, 50, 51, 81

www.ingramcontent.com/pod-product-compliance
Lightning Source LLC
Chambersburg PA
CBHW071134280326
41935CB00010B/1226